"Doctors Pulde and Lederman have written an easy-to-follow, four-week prescription to better health. Get it, read it, do it." —*Terry Mason, MD, chief medical officer for the Cook County Health and Hospitals System, Chicago, Illinois*

"Comprehensive, pragmatic, and beautifully simple. A big, plant-strong thumbs-up." —*Rip Esselstyn, former professional triathlete and author of* The Engine 2 Diet

"[This] powerful and practical four-step method provides readers with a GPS to health. We simply cannot afford to continue harming our bodies with food." —*Robert Ostfeld, MD, director of the Cardiac Wellness Program at Montefiore Medical Center*

"*Forks Over Knives* changed our lives! Eating plant-based is the one simple elegant thing that *everyone* can do to help clean up the environment and create a better planet where our children and grandchildren can thrive." —*Suzy Amis Cameron and James Cameron, environmental activists*

"Eating plants revolutionized every aspect of my life for the better. It worked for me and I promise it will work for you, too. So do yourself and your loved ones a favor and get this book!" —*Rich Roll, vegan ultra-endurance athlete and author of* Finding Ultra

"This life-changing book will empower you to feel better and live better." —*Gene Baur, founder of Farm Sanctuary*

"Yes, there's overwhelming scientific evidence that a whole-food, plant-based diet can save your life, but how do you actually do it? That's what *The Forks Over Knives Plan* is for!" —*Michael Greger, MD, founder of NutritionFacts.org*

"With *The Forks Over Knives Plan,* adopting a whole-food, plant-based lifestyle has never been easier or more delicious." —*Chef AJ, author of* Unprocessed

"This book is an absolute jewel! In just a few days, you can feel a growing confidence and excitement as you follow these stepping stones to the life you deserve." —*Doug Lisle, PhD, coauthor of* The Pleasure Trap

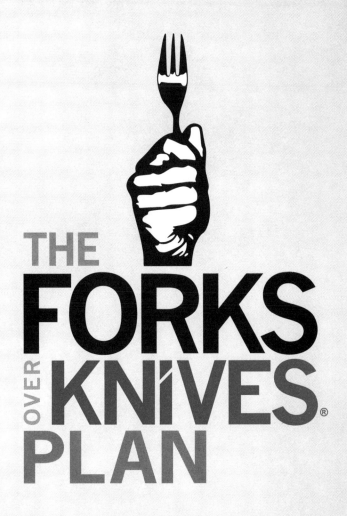

THE
FORKS
OVER KNIVES
PLAN

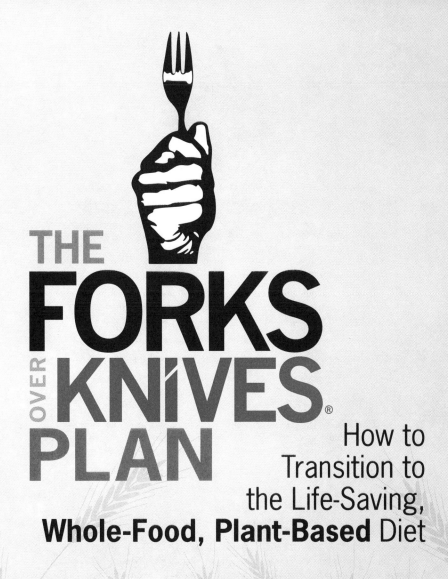

THE FORKS KNIVES PLAN

OVER

How to Transition to the Life-Saving, **Whole-Food, Plant-Based** Diet

Alona Pulde, MD, and Matthew Lederman, MD, with Marah Stets and Brian Wendel
Recipes by Darshana Thacker and Del Sroufe

ATRIA PAPERBACK

New York   London   Toronto   Sydney   New Delhi

ATRIA
PAPERBACK

An Imprint of Simon & Schuster, Inc.
1230 Avenue of the Americas
New York, NY 10020

This Atria Paperback edition January 2017

ATRIA PAPERBACK and colophon are registered trademarks of Simon & Schuster, Inc.

For information about special discounts for bulk purchases,
please contact Simon & Schuster Special Sales at
1-866-506-1949 or business@simonandschuster.com.

The Simon & Schuster Speakers Bureau can bring authors to your live event.
For more information or to book an event, contact the Simon & Schuster Speakers Bureau
at 1-866-248-3049 or visit our website at www.simonspeakers.com.

Interior design by Timothy Shaner, nightanddaydesign.biz

Manufactured in the United States of America

10

The Library of Congress has cataloged the Touchstone edition as follows:

Pulde, Alona.
The forks over knives plan : how to transition to the life-saving, whole-food,
plant-based diet / Alona Pulde, M.D. and Matthew Lederman, M.D. ; with Marah Stets and Brian Wendel.
pages   cm
"A Touchstone book."
1. Natural foods—Health aspects.   2. Veganism—Health aspects.   3. Cooking (Natural foods).
4. Vegan cooking.   5. Menus.   I. Lederman, Matt.   II. Stets, Marah.   III. Title.
RM237.55.P85   2014
641.5'636—dc23   2014009582

ISBN 978-1-4767-5329-4
ISBN 978-1-4767-5330-0 (pbk)
ISBN 978-1-4767-5331-7 (ebook)

We dedicate this book to the loves of our lives—

Kylee and Jordan—who remind us every day why we

do what we do and who make it all worthwhile

CONTENTS

Foreword

The most influential trend in medicine today, growing exponentially, is the emerging field of what is known as Lifestyle Medicine—lifestyle as *treatment,* not just prevention.

Doctors Alona Pulde and Matthew Lederman are extraordinary pioneers, leaders, and healers who represent the future of medicine. They are a new breed of doctors who integrate the most powerful medicine—good plant-based food—into the best of conventional medicine in how they treat their patients. They have empowered thousands of patients by practicing this way. Now, in *The Forks Over Knives Plan,* they will help many more understand that an important key to healing their bodies can be found in the foods that they eat. As they eloquently describe in this book, our bodies often have a remarkable capacity to begin healing if we focus on removing the main underlying *causes* of disease instead of just trying to eliminate the symptoms.

Many people tend to think of advances in medicine as high-tech and expensive, such as a new drug, laser, or surgical procedure. They often have a hard time believing that something as simple as diet and lifestyle changes can make such a powerful difference in our lives—but they often do. In our research, we've used high-tech, expensive, state-of-the-art scientific measures to prove the power of these simple, low-tech, and low-cost interventions.

For almost four decades, my colleagues and I at the nonprofit Preventive Medicine Research Institute and UCSF have conducted clinical research showing, for the first time, that a whole-food, plant-based diet (along with moving more, loving more, and stressing less) may reverse the progression of even severe coronary heart disease.

Many other doctors, such as those featured in the *Forks Over Knives* film (including Doctors Neal Barnard; Caldwell B. Esselstyn, Jr.; and John McDougall), have found similar results in their clinical practices and research.

My colleagues and I also found that these diet and lifestyle changes may stop or even reverse the progression of early-stage prostate cancer. We found that more than five hundred genes were changed in only three months—turning on genes that protect us and turning off genes that promote heart disease, type 2 diabetes, breast cancer, prostate cancer, and colon cancer, among others. Our latest research showed that even our telomeres get longer (the ends of our chromosomes that control aging); and as our telomeres get longer, our lives get longer. Thus, our genes are a predisposition, but our genes are not our fate.

All of these studies were published in the leading peer-reviewed medical journals and provide additional validity for the recommendations in this book. Based on this research, Medicare is now covering our lifestyle program, helping to create a new financially sustainable paradigm of health care rather than only sick care.

In each of these studies, we found that the more people changed their diet and lifestyle, the more they improved and the better they felt—at *any* age. It's not all or nothing. So, if you indulge yourself one day, just eat healthier the next. *The Forks Over Knives Plan* shows how to make this transition in a sustainable way.

The Forks Over Knives Plan is the right book at the right time. It can help transform your life for the better in sustainable ways. Because these underlying biological mechanisms are so dynamic, if you eat and live this way for just one week, you're likely to feel so much better so quickly that you'll find these are choices worth making—not from fear of dying but joy of living.

Dean Ornish, MD
Founder and president, Preventive Medicine Research Institute
Clinical professor of medicine, University of California, San Francisco
author of *The Spectrum* (and other books)
www.ornish.com

PART I

EATING THE FORKS OVER KNIVES WAY

I do not accept that I have to die of heart disease as my father did.

—Sylvia Cowe Nascimben, 68, retired project manager, Williamsville, NY

I no longer count calories and am losing weight naturally. I have more energy; I no longer have heartburn, colds, upset stomach.

—Laura McMullen, 64, retired, Federal Way, WA

You just get into a "groove." Whole-food, plant-based eating is just what you do—you don't even have to think about it.

—Nimisha Raja, 51, public relations/communications professional, Toronto ON, Canada

PART I

EATING THE FORKS OVER KNIVES WAY

**I do not accept that I have to die of
heart disease as my father did.**

—Sylvia Cowe Nascimben, 68, retired project manager, Williamsville, NY

**I no longer count calories and am losing weight
naturally. I have more energy; I no longer have
heartburn, colds, upset stomach.**

—Laura McMullen, 64, retired, Federal Way, WA

**You just get into a "groove." Whole-food,
plant-based eating is just what you do—you don't even
have to think about it.**

—Nimisha Raja, 51, public relations/communications professional,
Toronto ON, Canada

WHAT IS THE FORKS OVER KNIVES PLAN—**AND WHY WILL IT WORK FOR ME?**

CHAPTER 1

In the spring of 2009, we received a very interesting phone call. On the line was Brian Wendel, who said he was making a film on the power to prevent and treat chronic disease with a whole-food, plant-based diet. He turned to us because we were running our medical practice using this diet as a primary treatment. Brian wanted to show an audience how patients suffering from serious chronic conditions can, with relative ease and in a short time, turn around their difficult situations and achieve true health and vitality—just by eating well. Given our experience and training in lifestyle medicine, we were confident in this approach. We knew the power of this way of eating and were eager to help in whatever way we could to introduce its significant promise to a wide audience. And so without hesitation, we agreed. The film *Forks Over Knives* was released in theaters and on home video in 2011. The responses of audiences worldwide surpassed our best hopes for its reach and influence.

The food-as-medicine concept is now reaching millions of people and the movement is growing stronger each day. The movement's popularity is driven by one important factor: The lifestyle works! More and more people are learning that a diet based in fruits, vegetables, tubers, whole grains, and legumes makes all the difference when it comes to achieving good health . . . and the word is spreading in a big way.

Nearly five years after our involvement in the documentary, we are thrilled to have teamed up with Forks Over Knives again—this time to provide this four-week transition guide. In this book, we bring you the specifics of the Forks Over Knives philosophy and guide you through an A-to-Z transition so you can live the whole-food, plant-based way for a lifetime. Among other things, we detail what a whole-food, plant-based diet *is* and *is not*—and you'll see that this means you will be living on food that is not only healthy, but also hearty and satisfying. We show you how to survive and thrive on the foods you love—like pancakes, burritos, mashed potatoes, and lasagna—and at the same time, get all the nutrition you need.

People seek dietary changes for various reasons, whether it's to become healthier, lose weight, improve athletic performance, or just feel better. Regardless of the reasons for wanting a change, you are probably looking for a better result than you are getting now. Many diets fail because they tend to be nothing more than variations of the Standard American Diet. That is, they basically require a reshuffling of the same animal-based foods—oftentimes in order to meet target goals for certain individual nutrients, such as protein, calcium, or omega-3. They also tend to follow similar principles, such as counting calories or even purchasing supplements from the diet's author.

On the other hand, when you adopt the Forks Over Knives way of living, you will be trying something completely different. You will not be eating for single nutrients, counting calories, or buying supplements from us. Instead, you will simply focus on eating the whole, plant-based foods you enjoy. Though the food you'll eat is neither unfamiliar nor exotic, the *composition* of your plate of food will change substantially—so much so, in fact, that the lifestyle achieves something unlike anything else out there.

The hallmark of the whole-food, plant-based lifestyle is its unique ability to prevent, halt, and even treat chronic illness, such as heart disease and type 2 diabetes. The changes it can bring to your life are often rapid and measurable.

The ultimate goal of this program is simple: to leave you energized and free from debilitating chronic conditions so that you can spend less time in the doctor's office and more time with the people who are important to you, engaged in the activities you enjoy. This book will provide you with the tools you need to make it happen, including guidance and tips on stocking your house with good-tasting food; handling cravings; eating out; and dealing with social situations. Finally, we'll give you more than 100 recipes so that you have delicious meal and snack ideas literally at your fingertips.

As you'll learn from the pages that follow, we were once seeking dramatic changes in our own lives, and the lifestyle we discovered changed everything.

When you consult with your health care provider before you begin your transition, you should discuss with him or her any medication you are taking to manage a condition. Transitioning to a whole-food, plant-based diet may result, in possibly a very short time, in improvement in your condition for which you are taking medication, and your doctor may decide to adjust your medications and/or dosage. This is not because of a problem with the lifestyle. It is because your health may improve and as a result you may need a different dosage than you're taking now. It is very important that you and your doctor monitor the situation so you take only the amount of medication you need.

OUR STORIES

If you've seen the *Forks Over Knives* documentary, then you are already at least a little familiar with us, Dr. Alona Pulde and Dr. Matthew Lederman, and with what we do. We are two classically trained MDs who found traditional medicine lacking, given its emphasis on pills, drugs, and unnatural interventions. Instead, we've developed a food-first approach to practicing medicine. With this book, we'd like to share even more with you so that you, too, can start making changes in your diet, *today*. These changes will release you from the burdens of chronic disease, poor health, and a conventional medical system that in many cases offers little benefit and plenty of harm.

The four-week transition to the Forks Over Knives diet that we present in these pages has come about after years of treating our patients and seeing time and time again how food is truly the best medicine. Interestingly, if you had told either of us when we were first starting out that someday we would be prescribing food over medicine, we'd never have believed it. But we now believe this so fervently because we've seen the effects of this way of eating firsthand, in both our patients and in ourselves. It has changed the way we treat those in our care, and it's profoundly changed the way we think about medicine, food, disease, and health.

A brief editorial note before we introduce ourselves one at a time: This is the only time you'll hear from each of us individually. Speaking for ourselves we can more easily explain why each of us was seeking answers that conventional medicine could not provide and how the whole-food, plant-based diet became both our lifestyle and our cause. After this brief interlude, we will return to using our joint voice.

DR. PULDE'S STORY, IN HER OWN WORDS

For as long as I can remember, I have wanted to be a doctor, as evidenced early on by the teddy bears and dolls often lined up to see four-year-old Dr. Alona. I was as eager to help and heal those furry, stuffed paws way back then as I was excited to learn how to help and heal actual humans when I dove into the pre-med undergraduate program at UCLA many years later. Unfortunately, what I really learned there was that medicine had become a business more focused on making money by selling pills and procedures than on car-ing for and advocating for patients' rights and well-being. The doctor-patient relationship depicted best in the paintings of Norman Rockwell had disintegrated, as doctors were relegated to ten or fifteen minutes per patient and patients were restricted to just one complaint. It was no wonder these quick-fix methods were not producing successes and that patients were sinking deeper into their chronic illnesses, relying more and more on medications and "life-saving" procedures. I was devastated. This was *not* the medicine I had so anticipated practicing.

Fortunately, at the same time that I was coming to this disappointing realization, I was volunteering at a shelter for patients with HIV and AIDS. There I worked with an acupuncturist who taught me a completely different approach to medicine. She not only spent an hour with each patient, focusing on their needs, concerns, and ailments, but she treated them in a comprehensive manner that addressed their physical, mental, and emotional well-being. She didn't cure them of their disease, but she did alleviate a lot of the suffering associated with their illness as well as the side effects caused by their medications. Equally important, her patients felt heard, taken care of, and supported. *This* was the medicine I had always envisioned practicing, and so I pursued an education in Chinese medicine.

I spent four wonderful years at Emperor's College getting my degree in Traditional Chinese Medicine, which included courses in acupuncture and herbology. For the first time in my adult life, I was doing something I absolutely loved and completely believed in. I would have been happy to stay focused on traditional Chinese medicine for all of my career, except that my greatest mentor, Dr. Xiuling Ma, believed that the only way to truly provide comprehensive medical care to patients was to combine Eastern and Western medicines. She learned medicine this way and it was what made her so competent in her practice. And so I went back to school to get my medical degree.

Dr. Ma was absolutely correct that in order to be a comprehensive health care provider it is helpful to know, to understand, and to practice both Eastern and Western medicines. The knowledge and experience that I attained while in medical school are invaluable to my practice today—invaluable, but unfortunately also incomplete, as I discovered in a devastating way at the end of my second year of medical school, when my beloved father died suddenly.

With all my training and knowledge, I could not understand how a healthy man could suddenly die of a heart attack at age fifty-five. Yes, he had high cholesterol, but it was managed with cholesterol-lowering medication, and other than that, he was in terrific health. After all, we lived in a home that followed (for the most part) the Mediterranean diet. We ate tons of fruits, vegetables, and olive oil. We exercised regularly. We followed the recommended guidelines, hoping to reduce our cholesterol and fat intakes even more by eating chicken, turkey, and fish instead of beef and lamb; and our dairy intake was limited to occasional cheeses and ice cream. So, how could this happen? I was consumed with rage. What was this medicine—philosophy, pharmacology, and practice—worth if it couldn't allow a seemingly healthy and much-loved husband, father, and friend to live to a ripe old age? Obviously, I was missing something.

As luck, or maybe fate (thanks, Dad!), would have it, it was around this time that I met Matt, who had already discovered the answers I was looking for. He introduced me to the works of John McDougall, MD, T. Colin Campbell, PhD, and Caldwell Esselstyn, MD, among others. All at once, I was reawakened to a world where medicine was making a difference in people's lives. Patients were not only losing weight but were getting rid of their medications as they *reversed* their heart disease, *cured* their diabetes, and *reduced* their blood pressure and cholesterol.

How were they doing this? Through diet and lifestyle changes—specifically, by adopting a low-fat, whole-food, plant-based diet and eliminating animal products, oils, refined and processed foods, and bad habits like smoking. The more I read, the more I was enthralled, because for every argument I had—Where will I get my protein? Isn't olive oil good for you? What about calcium? Aren't chicken and fish healthy?—these doctors had an answer and the evidence to back it up. I evaluated the evidence only to find that they were right *every* time, although I really only needed to look at the success they were having with their patients to know what they were saying was true.

As with so many things in life, this was a bittersweet realization. Bitter because I wish I had known this information sooner, as it might have saved my dear father's life. But sweet, too, because I now have the opportunity to share this knowledge with the rest of my family and my friends, as well as you and your loved ones, in the hope that it will help you live the long, healthy, and happy life you deserve.

DR. LEDERMAN'S STORY, IN HIS OWN WORDS

I never really considered becoming anything other than a cardiologist, just like my father. Helping sick patients, participating in life-changing research, and being an educated resource to those in need drew me into this challenging profession. Unfortunately, after four years of medical school and three years of practicing medicine, I grew disillusioned and was ready to leave medicine altogether. I do not know what was to blame, whether it was the frustrations that come with a practice so driven by the pharmaceutical industry and the insurance industry or the simple fact that patients were not getting better despite my delivering the best care available. The medicine that I was practicing had very little to do with my original motivations to become a doctor.

Additionally, I felt lousy. I was physically ill. I couldn't go through a day without feeling awful. My stomach was my worst enemy. I was given the vague diagnosis of irritable bowel syndrome (IBS), and took pill after pill to reduce the stubborn symptoms. Nothing worked. My diet was healthy, according to modern medicine. I even removed lactose as much as possible, except when my cravings kicked in. My diet "hiccup" was a double barbecue bacon cheeseburger and fries followed by ice cream. "Every once in a while won't hurt," I thought. "Those foods are treats!"

I had already experienced my fair share of medical procedures and blood tests, looking for other potential causes of my escalating symptoms. I even went to integrative physicians and tried all sorts of alternative medications. I was considering yet another invasive procedure when my father reminded me of the risks involved. I was desperate, under the impression that more procedures would ultimately provide an answer. However, he challenged me to at least experiment with eliminating alcohol and junk foods before proceeding. The South Beach Diet I was on wasn't helping, but he wasn't sure what other diet to recommend. He was sure, however, that more medical care was clearly not the answer. Moreover, from a cardiologist's point of view, it couldn't hurt to at least stop the alcohol and fast food.

I committed *only* to doing some research. I went to the bookstore and read about nutrition and health, a topic overlooked in most medical schools. I was fascinated by the claims made by so many medical nutrition experts: reverse chronic disease, lose weight without dieting, lower cholesterol without medication, etc. "Craziness," I thought. "Likely just a bunch of medical quacks trying to sell an easy answer."

Thankfully, I was stubborn and determined to prove the medical nutrition experts wrong. I continued my research and exploration of medical journals and studies. I discovered that these experts told the truth, which was a hard truth for *me* to digest. I contacted Dr. John McDougall, one of the leading medical nutrition experts in the country, who has a successful practice in Northern California promoting plant-based nutrition as a medical strategy. Dr. McDougall kindly invited me to observe his practice, and I accepted.

I thank Dr. McDougall for reigniting my passion for medicine. His practice embodied my childhood understanding of what medicine should look and feel like. His patients were engaged in the process of becoming healthy and were empowered to make lifestyle changes. They were happy, excited, and thoroughly supported. As a result of following the McDougall program, his patients were reversing chronic diseases, losing weight, and seeing significantly improved blood test results. In my new excitement and enthusiasm, I decided that nutrition-based lifestyle medicine was the only way I could continue practicing medicine.

Somewhere in the process, I discovered that my stomach symptoms were undeniably related to my diet. Animal products (dairy, eggs, meat, fish), processed foods, and oil triggered painful reactions. Whole, plant-based foods were a joy to eat in comparison. It was an easy decision to hold off on further medical procedures and instead opt to continue with my nutrition experiment.

I committed to eating a whole-food, plant-based diet. Unfortunately, these foods were hard to come by, even in health-conscious Los Angeles. Most vegan restaurants doused their food in oils and depended heavily on processed foods (there were commercial meat substitutes galore in their kitchens). Additionally, despite my abilities to perform complex medical procedures, I could barely figure out how to turn on my stove. At first I ate simple plant-based whole foods: oats, rice, beans, fruits, and vegetables. I ate what I could cook. But after about a week, my willpower ran out. I felt miserably deprived. In a moment of frustration, after passing my favorite fast-food drive-thru, I succumbed to a double barbecue bacon cheeseburger and fries. The resulting pain reminded me that this food is far from harmless.

I committed to trying whole, plant-based foods again, only this time I knew I needed to arm myself with the tools to succeed. If eating out was not a regular option, I needed to learn how to cook. I started slowly and learned to cook one recipe at a time. I learned how to be forgiving, as I cooked some meals I wouldn't wish upon my worst enemy. Each "failure" was a new lesson. Each lesson helped me reach my ultimate goal of feeling healthy and happy. Real failure was just not an option.

Without even trying, I lost weight. At 6 feet tall, I weighed 195 pounds when I started my new diet and lifestyle, and I am now a lean 180 pounds. My stomach troubles are also under control, so long as I follow a diet filled with whole, plant-based foods. My blood test results are impressive. But, more than all of that, I am happy. I enjoy what I eat, and I love that I am pain-free and finally have some control over my health.

Despite my success, I received a lot of criticism and judgment from my medical colleagues, my peers, and even my family. It's been a hard journey. I am aware of how crazy my claims may sound to newcomers. In fact, I had those exact same thoughts until I experimented on myself. But trust me—I'm a doctor! (Actually, in all seriousness, never trust anyone who tells you to trust them simply because they are a doctor. Trust how you feel, the results you see, the happiness you derive, and, hopefully, unbiased science.)

SHARING THE MESSAGE WITH YOU

We spent the early years in our careers working within a medical system focused on alleviating symptoms more than on fixing the core problems. We found an approach that brings about something far more satisfying and lasting, and we've seen what it did in our own lives. Furthermore, we have studied and researched what most doctors don't ever think about: the relationship between food and the human body. Armed with facts, research, and healthy recipes, we have helped our patients—not to mention family, friends, and colleagues—understand how to transition to optimum health. We are enormously grateful to our mentors and to each other, for we now walk this path absolutely united (both professionally and personally) as physicians focused on being true patient advocates. Ultimately, we refuse to recommend anything other than the safest, most effective, evidence-based medicine available.

With this four-week guide we are providing you with a road map to health. We will show you how in just one month you can transition to an entirely whole-food, plant-based diet—meal by meal, week by week. By the end of these four weeks it will be clear how what you eat affects your body and why this way of eating is the best way to stay strong and achieve optimum health. The decision of what to do with this evidence and whether you follow this map is entirely up to you. Once you read this book, you will have all the information you need to be fully armed for success. You can decide to think of this as an overwhelming lifestyle change, or you can decide that you want to take control of your health and run with it. Either way, you are choosing how to live the rest of your life.

GETTING PERSONAL

Whenever I am feeling down, or start to think my choices are extreme or radical, I turn to online support, or open a book, to remind myself. What I am doing is making a difference. I am not only making choices to increase my longevity, but I am ensuring a better quality of life for myself by feeling good each day that I have.
—Jodie Plummer, 40, medical office administrator, Nottawa, Ontario, Canada

My life is, well, better—in every way! The first things I noticed were my boost in energy and the enhanced taste sensations of my taste buds. After cutting out animal foods and cutting down on processed foods, fruits and vegetables began to explode with flavor I had never experienced before. I also cook (well) now—and I enjoy it! Before: a bowl of cereal, a grilled cheese sandwich, a chicken breast with some salt and pepper. Now: chickpea curry, monster kale salads, sweet potato polenta stacks, homemade veggie burgers, and much more.
—Steven Todd Smith, 30, Reiki master teacher, life nutrition coach, FOK community manager, Los Angeles, CA

This is not a diet. It is just a change in lifestyle and approaching food differently—it's a different way of thinking. . . . Another woman that I work with and I are trying to set up a monthly meeting group—gathering people that are on this same journey, so we can share thoughts and ideas.
—Laura Hoepfner, 63, teacher, Appleton, WI

My husband and I have learned about all sorts of foods we never knew about before, and enjoy the greater variety. Both of us have experienced improved blood work (labs), weight loss, increased energy, and less joint pain.

—Kathy Mode, 50, retired, Daytona Beach, FL

Once the processed foods, meat, dairy, and other garbage were removed from my diet, the taste buds came alive and vegetables tasted so much better than they used to.

—Jamie Lasee, 39, recreation director, Fond du Lac, WI

When I think about how miserable I was before, how sick I was, it's amazing to me how much simple dietary changes have changed everything about the quality of my life.

—Suzanne Schier-Happell, 37, college professor, Columbus, OH

LET FOOD BE THY MEDICINE:
The Science Behind a
Whole-Food, Plant-Based Diet

We will begin the four-week transition in chapter 4. First, we want to show you how a whole-food, plant-based diet will actually improve your health, as opposed to the procedures and prescriptions of conventional medicine, which in most cases only improve the indicators of disease—without significantly helping to prevent or eliminate the disease itself. In this chapter, we demonstrate why letting food be your medicine is the smartest step you can take to ensure your excellent health for a lifetime.

Let's face it: Americans are sick, tired, and overmedicated. Every fifty-three seconds someone in the United States dies of heart disease, which, as the nation's number-one killer, claims about 600,000 lives per year.[1] Cancer, now the second leading cause of death, takes the lives of more than 1,500 people per day.[2] Meanwhile, nearly 10 percent of the population has diabetes[3]; and our children are getting sicker, as indicated by the startling fact that obesity has more than doubled in children and tripled in adolescents in the past thirty years.[4] We have turned to the medical system for help, and it has delivered medication in a big way: Nearly 70 percent of Americans are on at least one prescription drug, more than 50 percent take two, and 20 percent are on five or more prescription drugs.[5] Despite the billions of dollars being spent on phar-maceuticals, the needle almost never moves downward on the rates of chronic disease, and people still feel lousy and sick.

Health statistics aren't just about numbers on a page or data on a statisti-cian's ledger. These are our mothers, fathers, siblings, and children. These are our friends. The health crisis is taking a real toll on our daily lives, profoundly affecting the personal happiness and productivity of millions of us every sin-gle day.

There is good news, though. Research is revealing with greater certainty that we understand the main cause of this epidemic: an American diet that derives more than 90 percent of what we eat from animal-based and processed foods.[6] *Understanding the cause means there's hope!* The research tells us that if we change to an entirely different *way* of eating, we can dramatically alter our health destiny.[7]

Modern pioneers like T. Colin Campbell, PhD; Caldwell Esselstyn, MD; Dean Ornish, MD; John McDougall, MD; Neal Barnard, MD; and others are leading the charge. Thanks to these doctors and researchers, along with an emerging body of scientific evidence from all corners, we now know that a whole-food, plant-based diet is more powerful at preventing and treating chronic diseases than any medication or procedure. We are so convinced by the evidence that we believe if this diet came in a pill, it would be heralded on the front pages of newspapers and magazines around the world for its effectiveness.

There is a movement under way as hundreds of thousands of people, if not more, are trying the whole-food, plant-based lifestyle for themselves and finding great success. We have personally seen remarkable results in our own medical practice, not to mention experienced it in our own lives. Here are just a few of the significant life-changing results you may expect:

■ **Prevent and reverse the leading chronic ailments.** A whole-food, plant-based diet can prevent, halt, and even reverse heart disease[8] and diabetes.[9] Other diseases that are also positively impacted by this type of diet include: high cholesterol, high blood pressure, obesity, and overall mortality.[10] Cancer is also significantly affected by this diet. In fact, the foods that make up this diet are the exact same foods that were recommended in the first "surviving cancer" dietary recommendations.[11] There is also evidence that a plant-based diet may reduce the risk of diverticular disease, gallstones, rheumatoid arthritis, gout, and kidney disease.[12] Furthermore, after switching to a plant-based diet, people routinely report experiencing or seeing in others improvements in a range of ailments, including osteoporosis, arthritis, headaches, acne, asthma, sexual dysfunction, reflux, lupus, inflammatory bowel disease, constipation, irritable bowel syndrome, dementia, Alzheimer's, multiple sclerosis, infertility, insomnia, and sleep apnea. They even find themselves experiencing fewer or less intense colds, viruses, and allergies.

■ **Reach your ideal weight.** Our friend Doug Lisle likes to point out that humans and their domesticated pets are the only earthly creatures that suffer from being overweight and obese . . . in spite of the fact that we're also the only creatures who practice portion control! Why is this the case? It's simple. All of the other animals on earth are eating foods that are appropriate for their species. If we also eat the foods that are appropriate for our species—whole, plant-based foods—then we, too, will be able to eat without portion control and will naturally reach a comfortable weight. (We'll talk more about this in our discussion of calorie density and body weight on page 30.)

■ **Improve mental clarity.** Eating a whole-food, plant-based diet improves cognitive function and protects against dementia and Alzheimer's disease.[13] Most people experience greater clarity of thought, improved ability to concentrate, and better memory.

■ **Experience only *positive* effects, not "side effects."** Perhaps you have chosen to transition to a plant-based diet to reverse heart disease or reduce your diabetes medications, but now that you're here, you can see that you're about to welcome into your life an abundance of positive effects. These can include better mood, sounder sleep, improved bowel function, and more vibrant skin. You will have more energy to do the things you love, like playing with your children or grandchildren, biking, gardening, walking, swimming. You may even *want* to exercise more. By contrast, as we'll discuss in more detail a little later, medical procedures and medications can have all sorts of major unintended negative consequences.

■ **Have a sense of well-being and empowerment.** *You* are in control of your health. You do not have to settle for compromised health or believe that you are destined to succumb to chronic disease. You can live with less fear that a heart attack can happen at any time or that you will be struck by the same chronic ailment from which other members of your family have suffered.

■ **Save time and money.** Whether you have health insurance or not, you will likely have to pay out of pocket for at least some of your health care expenses if you are sick. Fewer trips to the doctor and fewer procedures and pills equal more time and money you can spend in other areas of your life.

"IMPROVING YOUR NUMBERS" ISN'T ENOUGH: WE WANT YOU TO BE HEALTHY!

It's not unusual for a person who is sick to go to the doctor, who very often prescribes medications to treat whatever ails the patient. In the case of conditions such as high cholesterol or high blood pressure, these medications will usually improve the patient's elevated numbers, but the medications do not address the underlying sickness. Further, improved numbers can lead to a false sense of security about the condition, which can continue to wreak havoc on the patient's health even while the "numbers" look good.

This is largely the way of modern medicine. Doctors are focused on fixing the indicators of disease and not the disease itself. And that's folly, pure and simple. Consider what it would be like if we treated our car in the same way: If the "check engine" light were on, we would disable the light and think we'd fixed the engine. That would never happen, right? And yet consider heart disease and cholesterol for a moment: How many doctors and pharmaceutical companies speak about high cholesterol as if it's a disease in and of itself? It's not. High cholesterol is an *indicator* of disease. The disease is sick arteries. Statins will improve your cholesterol numbers, but they will do little for those arteries.

Achieving good biometrics, or "numbers," through healthy living is very different than achieving those same numbers through medication. Let's look at one example and see how a good biometric from healthy living compares to one from medication. Consider the case of blood pressure and risk of heart attack and stroke for a man aged 40 to 59. If the man has high blood pressure and significantly lowers it with medication, he will still have a 20 percent *higher* chance of having one of these major cardiac events than someone who has a normal blood pressure from healthy living.[14] The reason for this is simple: High blood pressure is an indicator that the cardiovascular system is clogged, and the blood pressure medication does little to address this problem.

As medical doctors, it is incumbent upon us to let our patients know about the safest and most effective treatments. In this case, we want you to unclog your arteries—not merely shut off the indicator light with medicine. And the research informs us how to do this: a low-fat, whole-food, plant-based lifestyle. Virtually all of our patients will achieve a normal blood pressure—and more important, *healthy arteries*—when they adopt this way of eating. Similarly, if it's high blood sugar from type 2 diabetes, or acid reflux, or any one of a number of chronic conditions, our goal is the same: Make the *system* as healthy as possible, so it doesn't produce symptoms in the first place. And a healthy system just plain makes you *feel* better than a medicated one.

PILLS AND PROCEDURES HAVE BIG PROBLEMS

In modern-day health care, medication and procedures are usually the first line of defense. As we just discussed, meds can improve symptoms or biometrics, but they do little or nothing to resolve the underlying problem. Sometimes medication and procedures may improve your chances of avoiding a health catastrophe, although in most instances, only slightly. Meanwhile, the tools of modern health care that are intended to help us can in fact cause serious harm, and the downside of going down this road should be carefully considered by the patient and doctor. Just to be clear, we are *not* saying that medication and procedures should always be avoided—of course they are *sometimes* justified. But you, the patient, should be well aware of the potential benefits and risks. In our research, we often find that common diagnostic tests and medical treatments yield benefits that are so minimal or that affect so few people, that any plusses are far outweighed by the potential for damage. Consider these medications and procedures, along with some of their potential harmful effects:

- **Blood pressure medications.** Increased risk of heart attack, stroke, and cancer.[15]

- **Cholesterol-lowering medications, including statins.** Cognitive dysfunction, diabetes, falls, muscle pain, and long-term liver damage.[16]

- **Bypass surgery.** Brain damage and cognitive dysfunction.[17]

- **Diabetes medications.** Some medications increase the risk of heart attack and fracture risk.[18]

- **Chemotherapy.** Extremely toxic and with severe side effects, including hair loss, nausea, vomiting, and nerve damage.[19]

- **Mammograms.** False positives and over-diagnosis lead to unnecessary radiation treatment, chemotherapy, and mastectomies.[20]

- **Bone density scans.** Erroneous diagnosis of osteopenia and osteoporosis leads to unnecessary treatments with severe side effects, such as bone death.[21]

- **PSA testing.** Over-diagnosis leads to unnecessary treatments that can cause impotence and incontinence.[22]

Ironically, or tragically, these medications and procedures are used to treat ailments that are mostly preventable, and often reversible, with diet and lifestyle. A whole-food, plant-based diet can give you the freedom to avoid unnecessary procedures, ineffective treatments, and expensive pills. *You* can accomplish a healthy life far better with your own food choices than a doctor can with medical treatment. The power is in *your* hands!

EATING RUNS IN FAMILIES:
MAKE HEALTH, NOT GENETICS, YOUR DESTINY

You may recall from *Forks Over Knives* how a study of a broad cross section of the Chinese population in the 1970s found death rates from certain cancers to be highly variable from region to region. In fact, though the people were ethnically similar, cancer mortality rates differed by as much as four hundred–fold depending on where in the country people lived.[23] Such high variation among ethnically similar people indicates something different than genetics is at play here; and indeed, the comprehensive China-Oxford-Cornell Project that followed implicated dietary factors, specifically those relating to the consumption of animal foods, as being significantly associated with Western type diseases.[24] Other studies have had results consistent with these findings, including one published in 1981 that found that no more than 3 to 4 percent of cancer cases are attributable to genetics.[25]

If you have heart disease or diabetes and your parents had it, the primary common link is not your genetics, but that you all likely ate and still eat the same food. The problem with these kinds of chronic ailments rests primarily in the fact that animal products and oils have been eaten across the generations. If you change the way you eat, you have a good chance of changing your destiny. This is why you may have heard it said that genetics loads the gun but environment pulls the trigger. In other words, for most conditions, genetics may play a small role by making us more *predisposed* to a given condition, but it is your diet and lifestyle that are the most important factors in ultimately determining whether you will actually suffer from a chronic disease or not.

HELPING YOU REACH YOUR GOAL

Most of the patients we have worked with want much more than to feel merely a little bit better. They want improved vitality, vibrancy, and disease-free living. They want more time and energy to enjoy with their families or to be more active or more productive in their work. We are confident you want this too; after all, you have chosen to read this book. In the *Forks Over Knives* documentary, the filmmakers asked, is there a solution to chronic disease that is "so comprehensive, yet so straightforward, that it's mind-boggling that more of us haven't taken it seriously"? The answer, we believe, is an emphatic *yes*—with the solution, of course, being a whole-food, plant-based lifestyle. But don't take our word for it. Dive in and experience the benefits for yourself!

GETTING PERSONAL

I was tired of feeling like crap! I was always fatigued, felt depressed often, and had doctors telling me it had nothing to do with my diet and I just needed to take some anxiety meds and call it good. I just knew in my heart that it was what I was feeding my body, and once I decided to start searching out what I needed to do to get my body back to health, *everything* changed!

—Amanda Pettera, 33, dental assistant/homemaker, Mesa, AZ

I work with the general public in a health-related field. I see how many medications people are on because of their weight and inactivity. I see how many dollars are spent monthly on drugs like Lipitor, Qsymia, and breathing medications. It saddens me to know how easy it is to be healthy and live simply when these people are obviously struggling.

—Danielle Eckerle, 28, pharmacy technician, Corvallis, OR

I went vegan while undergoing chemotherapy and noticed a huge change! What used to take me two weeks to recover from a treatment, would now only take two days! I had so much more energy. I also felt lighter in my body (and mind), not that heavy feeling I used to get from eating animal products. And my hair started growing back!

—Hayley Holroyd, 32, artist, Vancouver, BC, Canada

Everything is different! I'm very much still transitioning, but my skin, energy, sleep, and mood have all improved. I never expected how much changing how I eat could affect my ability to manage stress, either—it's like a weight has been lifted. I also feel like I'm more compassionate as a human being. One of the most noticeable differences is that I have not had a single cold since beginning this journey a year ago. I normally get several colds a year and at least one bout of bronchitis and/or pneumonia. That change is *amazing*!

—Faith Henry, 30, educational platform and marketing manager, Biddeford, ME

I've had people ask me if I'm still sticking to my "diet." I tell them it's not a diet, it's a lifestyle, and that I can never go back to eating the way I did before because I can't "unknow" all the things I now know.

—Pam Cowperthwaite, 48, teacher, Carson City, NV

When I discovered that many athletes had started to go on plant-based diets, I decided to give it a try. I actually found it easy to give up meat. I was really surprised. I also found it easy to adapt to eating more fruits and vegetables. I didn't expect that.

—Stephen Bottiau, 37, teacher, Angoulême, France

I expected to struggle but have not. The thirty days from when I started was timed to end on Thanksgiving dinner so I could have my favorite meal of the year— but we ended up having vegetable lasagna instead.

—Atania Gilmore, 55, program manager
for a contract manufacturer, Spokane, WA

THE FORKS OVER KNIVES LIFESTYLE: **How Can Eating *More* Lead to Weight Loss and Better Health?**

Now that you've learned the powerful benefits of whole-food, plant-based eating, the next step is to harness that power for yourself. We need to cover a few basics first, and then you'll be ready to dive right in to your own four-week transition in chapter 4.

WHAT IS A WHOLE-FOOD, PLANT-BASED DIET?

A whole-food, plant-based diet is centered on whole, unrefined, or minimally refined plants. It's a diet based on fruits, vegetables, tubers, whole grains, and legumes; and it excludes or minimizes meat (including chicken and fish), dairy products, and eggs, as well as highly refined foods like bleached flour, refined sugar, and oils.

We know that's a mouthful! We'll get into the details of what you will eat and what your meals will look like a little later. In the meantime, just rest assured that you'll be eating in a way that people have thrived on for thousands of years. We believe that you will find—as we do—that the diet and foods are very tasty and satisfying. Following are the food categories from which you'll eat, along with a few examples from each. These include the ingredients you'll be using to make familiar dishes, such as pizza, mashed potatoes, lasagna, and burritos:

- **Fruit:** mangoes, bananas, grapes, strawberries, blueberries, oranges, cherries, etc.

- **Vegetables:** lettuce, collard greens, broccoli, cauliflower, kale, carrots, etc.

- **Tubers and starchy vegetables:** potatoes, yams, yucca, winter squash, corn, green peas, etc.

- **Whole grains:** millet, quinoa, barley, rice, whole wheat, oats, etc.

- **Legumes:** kidney beans, chickpeas, lentils, lima beans, cannellini beans, black beans, etc.

Now that you know generally what sorts of foods you'll be eating, let's delve further into what the diet is—and what it most definitely is *not*.

A Whole-Food, Plant-Based Diet Is *Not* a Diet of Vegetables

You may have heard that people living this way eat lots of spinach, kale, and collard greens, and that this is, in fact, the primary basis for many of the meals. You may even think we live *only* on leafy and raw vegetables. However, nothing could be further from the truth.

While leafy vegetables are an important part of the whole-food, plant-based diet, they are a very poor calorie, i.e., energy, source. We would need to eat almost *16 pounds* of cooked kale to get 2,000 calories of food! We certainly don't eat this way, and we wouldn't blame you for thinking it sounds crazy—we think so, too! In fact, *it is virtually impossible to get enough calories from leafy vegetables alone to form a sustainable diet.* Perhaps the most common reason for failure in this lifestyle is that people actually try to live on leafy vegetables alone. If you try to live on these vegetables, you become deficient in calories. Not eating enough calories leads you to feel hungry, which over time may result in decreased energy, feelings of deprivation, cravings, and even binges. These issues are *not* caused by switching to a plant-based diet—rather, they are all related to not eating enough.

Don't get us wrong: We certainly recommend you eat generous amounts of leafy vegetables. But these are complementary foods that you eat regularly. They are *not* the energy source on your food plate.

So if leafy vegetables aren't the basis of a whole-food, plant-based lifestyle, what *is*?

Starch-Based Foods and Fruit Form the Basis of the Whole-Food, Plant-Based Diet

In America most of us are accustomed to building our dinner plate around meat. This will change with your new lifestyle. The center of your plate is now going to be the starch-based comfort foods most of us have always loved, but that have long been relegated to side dishes or stigmatized because of a misperception that they are "unhealthy." Yet these are the foods that people around the world have thrived on for generations: tubers like potatoes and sweet potatoes; starchy vegetables like corn and peas; whole grains like brown rice, millet, quinoa, and buckwheat; and legumes like chickpeas, black beans, kidney beans, and lima beans.

They may be prepared a bit differently—leaving out oil and dairy, for example—but most of them will nonetheless be familiar. Those that aren't may become delightful new discoveries you'll make as part of embarking on your new lifestyle. They come in the form of delicious dishes like Sweet Potato Lasagna (page 213), Mashed Potatoes and Gravy (page 180), Tuscan White

Bean Burgers (page 166), Easy Thai Noodles (page 237), Lima Bean Soup (page 205), Shepherd's Pot Pie (page 224), Black Bean and Rice Burritos (page 158), Polenta Curry (page 250), and Spicy French Fries (page 185). In addition to starch-based foods, you can enjoy as much whole fruit as you like.

NO MORE EATING FOR SINGLE NUTRIENTS . . . FOCUS ON THE "PACKAGE" AND THE FOODS YOU ENJOY

The idea of eating a particular food for one nutrient is pervasive in our culture. We have been led to believe we should eat meat for protein, dairy for calcium, fish for omega-3 fatty acids, and even tomatoes for lycopene, among many others. This sort of thinking is misguided and has caused grave harm to human health. The quest for protein, for example, has steered us toward meat consumption. In this quest, we not only consume protein in *excess* of our needs, but also many harmful substances like dietary cholesterol that are only present in animal foods.

No food is a single nutrient, and we should never think of foods in that way. Any given food has *countless* nutrients. What matters most is the overall nutrient profile, i.e., the whole package. Whole, plant-based foods contain *all* the essential nutrients (with the exception of vitamin B_{12}*), and in proportions that are more consistent with human needs than animal-based or processed foods. So our question is really this: Why waste *any* of what we eat on inferior packages? As long as—over time—we choose a variety of whole, plant-based foods, we will easily meet all of our nutritional needs.

Even on this diet, people sometimes tend to worry about eating a certain type of green vegetable for calcium, beans for protein, nuts for fat, and so on. We ask you to let go of that kind of thinking. The most important thing in this lifestyle is to choose the whole, plant-based food you enjoy most.

---

* We discuss vitamin B_{12} on page 37. Sometimes vitamin D is considered a nutrient, although it's really a hormone. It's generally not found in sufficient amounts in food and is best obtained by exposing the skin to sunlight in safe amounts. See page 37 for more information.

Whole, Plant-Based Food Will Provide the Best "Package" of Nutrients

When eating fruits, vegetables, tubers, whole grains, and legumes to comfortable satiation, you will get superior nutrition without also getting all the unhealthy elements present in animal-based and highly processed foods. Among other things, you will effortlessly consume:

- **A nutrient profile consistent with human needs.** All whole foods contain carbohydrates, protein, and fat. These are the macronutrients, which are the source of virtually all calories, or energy. Different foods, however, contain each of these in different proportions. The foods you eat on a whole-food, plant-based diet will most easily get you to a healthy carbohydrate, protein, and fat ratio, which lies somewhere in the range of 80/10/10. We discuss each macronutrient in the chapters that follow.

- **Lower-calorie-density foods that will leave you neither underweight nor overweight.** Whole, plant-based foods in general are significantly lower in calories per pound (calorie density) than animal products and processed food. Higher-calorie-density foods lead to excessive calorie consumption and overweight bodies. Many chronic diseases are caused by the same foods that result in being overweight or obese. (We explain calorie density and how it affects body weight on page 30.)

- **A sufficient amount of vitamins and minerals.** Every vitamin or mineral you need to thrive is present in a whole-food, plant-based diet in amounts and proportions consistent with our needs. The only exceptions are vitamin B_{12} and vitamin D, which we discuss on page 37.

- **Dietary fiber.** Fiber plays a key role in signaling to our brain that we have eaten enough and is also an essential part of digestion, normal colon function, and binding and removing toxins that would otherwise be reabsorbed into the body. Animal foods do not contain any dietary fiber, so we must get it from whole plant foods.

- **No cholesterol.** We do not need to consume cholesterol in our diets because our bodies can make all that we need. Avoiding dietary cholesterol is a great way to decrease our risk of developing heart disease. Excess cholesterol is involved in the thickening and hardening of arteries, or atherosclerosis, which leads to serious problems, such as heart attacks and strokes. Animal foods, even the low-fat varieties, contain cholesterol.

UNDERSTANDING CALORIE DENSITY AND HOW IT AFFECTS BODY WEIGHT

A calorie is a measure of the energy in food. Specifically, a calorie is the approximate amount of energy needed to raise the temperature of one gram of water by one degree Celsius. Even if this exact definition is new to you, you likely understand, as most people do, that if we increase the number of calories in our diet, we will gain weight. Conversely, if we eat less of them, then the pounds will come off. People's understanding of this has led many to read labels and seek out foods with limited calories.

We must consume a certain quantity of food at each meal before our stomach stretches enough to signal satiety. The problem with decreasing calories is that the only way to do this on the Standard American Diet is to actually decrease the quantity of food that we eat. Consuming this smaller volume leads to feelings of hunger, as our body wants to fill the void with more food. Usually, over time hunger pangs win out over our willpower, and we consume more high-calorie foods until our stomach has stretched sufficiently to signal satiety. And yet many diet plans continue to espouse the view that we should count calories, even though doing so is neither a pleasant nor, for most people, effective way to control weight.

One of the major advantages of the whole-food, plant-based diet is that you will not need to count calories or practice portion control. Plant-based foods have a lot more bulk because they contain more fiber and water than the standard American "diet" foods. This bulk takes up more space, so our stomachs end up stretching sufficiently to shut off hunger signals despite our having consumed fewer calories overall. As such, a whole-food, plant-based diet is the only way to eat to feel full while also consuming fewer calories.

While we don't recommend that you count calories, we do think it's helpful to understand *calorie density,* which is different than simply *calories.* Calorie density is the number of calories in a given weight of food. We tend to express this as calories per pound. Certain foods have more calories packed into them pound for pound. For example, as shown in the list below, leafy vegetables contain 100 to 200 calories per pound while oil contains 4,000 calories per pound. If you are eating a diet based on fruits, vegetables, tubers, whole grains, and legumes (and you are not relying solely on vegetables), then the meals you consume will average a calorie density of approximately 550 (or fewer) calories per pound. Note that it is okay to include some foods above this calorie density as long as the average is about 550 or below. Eating in this range will provide both the correct number of calories and the appropriate volume of food needed to properly and timely signal your body that it has had enough to eat. This will help you reach or maintain a healthy body weight.

If you generally consume foods with a high calorie density, they will take up less space in your stomach and you will tend to consume more calories than you need in order to feel full. This will, as you might guess, lead to a person being overweight or obese. See the figure on page 33, which you might recognize from the *Forks Over Knives* documentary; it shows how equal calorie counts for different foods do not translate to equal quantities of those foods, nor do they provide the same amount of satiation. You can see that 500 calories of plant foods provides much more bulk than 500 calories of processed foods or oil. This is a big reason why those foods cause us to overeat—they simply aren't as filling!

While it's common for people to believe that body weight is primarily determined by our ability to control portions and "walk away from the table," the reality is quite different. Body weight is more a function of food choices. The more calorie-dense, or concentrated, the foods we choose, the more likely we will be to find ourselves overweight. (We can also begin to understand how the problems with societal obesity are not about people becoming less disciplined over time, but more about the food supply becoming more concentrated and calorie-dense.) In order to reach a comfortable body weight, we simply need to choose the right foods—which is much easier and more effective than counting calories and controlling our portion sizes. If we choose the whole, plant-based foods that are healthy for us, our body's natural mechanisms for controlling weight will take care of the rest.

Eating Until You Are Satisfied Is Important on a Whole-Food, Plant-Based Diet

If you enjoy eating like we do, this will be good news. The lower calorie density of whole, plant-based foods *requires* you to eat until you are comfortably satisfied in order to make the diet work. Portion control, in fact, can lead to insufficient calorie intake. So in order to succeed, you will need to really eat! In fact, you will likely have to *increase* the volume of food in your diet.

If you have long been used to eating a steak and a baked potato for dinner, you cannot expect to drop the steak and have just one baked potato as your meal. If you eat a meal of plain baked potatoes, you might require two, three, or more. After a period of adjustment, you might notice you need to have second or third helpings of, say, sweet potato stew or vegetable shepherd's pie in order to feel satisfied. Until you figure out this balance for yourself, you might also need snacks during the day. Don't try to resist eating additional low calorie density food when you are hungry or you may unknowingly be harming your chances of success with this program. In general, whole, plant-based foods won't make you gain weight as long as you are eating an *average* calorie density of 550 (or fewer) calories per pound.

The important lesson here is that you should begin to trust your own hunger and satiety signals. You're most likely used to calories being packed into

Satiation with Fewer Calories

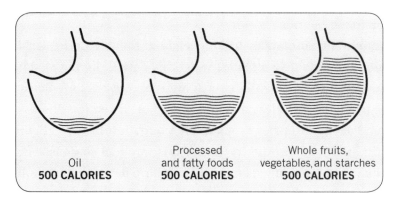

| Oil **500 CALORIES** | Processed and fatty foods **500 CALORIES** | Whole fruits, vegetables, and starches **500 CALORIES** |

small volumes, so you'll need to grow accustomed to new, larger quantities of food in order to succeed in the long run. With patience, it will work, and we are confident you will find this a very gratifying part of your new lifestyle.

Calorie Density to Find a Preferred Weight

Even on a whole-food, plant-based diet, we can adjust our average calorie density by lowering or increasing it to find a preferred body weight. So if weight loss is your primary goal, lowering the calorie density of your meals will help the weight come off faster. You can see from the chart on page 34 that fruit, for example, has a calorie density of 200 to 400 calories per pound, while whole grains, such as cooked oats, clock in at 400 to 500 calories per pound. This means that having a breakfast of fruit or a single bowl of oatmeal loaded with a variety of fruit will have a lower calorie density than several bowls of plain oatmeal. Further, a couple of bowls of oatmeal will have a lower calorie density than the same portion of whole wheat toast, because the latter is more processed and therefore has higher calorie density.

You can also try this trick for more rapid weight loss. For any meal, you can begin with foods that have a lower calorie density. For example, try beginning a meal with some fruit or a big salad. You can also add more vegetables to your plate and have them before or with your denser main course. These small measures will add low calorie density with high volume, which will leave you satiated on fewer calories.

One important note about losing weight through calorie density: Some people think they can lose the most weight by eating the fewest calories, living off raw and leafy vegetables (which are the lowest-calorie-density foods). While it is true that you'll lose a lot of weight quickly eating this way, you will not consume enough calories to maintain energy levels or to eliminate cravings. We find that people who try eating this way feel so deprived that they "fall off the wagon" and binge on the most calorie-dense and unhealthy foods. In other words, they seesaw from romaine lettuce to chili cheeseburgers rather than living comfortably on potatoes. So feel free to add in lots of raw and leafy veggies, but don't forget to eat the foods that satisfy.

Calorie Density for Common Foods

Here is the approximate calorie density (calories per pound) for a variety of common foods.[26] It's best to eat a whole-food, plant-based diet that *averages* approximately 550 calories per pound.

Raw and leafy vegetables	70–200
Fruits	200–400
Tubers and starchy vegetables	300–400
Whole grains	400–500
Legumes	500–600
Whole wheat pasta, cooked	550
Avocado	750
Whole wheat bread	1,150
Meat	1,200
Pure sugar	1,800
Chocolate	2,200
Nuts and seeds	2,600
Oils	4,000

Calorie Density After Your Workout

After a workout, the hunger drive is likely to be very strong as your calorie needs will be higher. In these moments, richer foods may be appealing. However, we recommend big quantities of low-calorie-density foods instead of high-calorie-density foods. The kind of foods you should be eating doesn't change based on your activity level, only the quantity does. So after the run or bicycle ride, or the hour in the gym, head home and eat a big bowl of oatmeal, some rice and beans, or a meal of seasoned potatoes. High-performance athletes in particular will need to make sure they are eating sufficiently large volumes. They may also need to consume some amount of higher-calorie-density, whole, plant-based foods.

AVOID SUPPLEMENTS—EXCEPT FOR VITAMIN B$_{12}$

The relationship between whole food and the human body is very intricate and has come about as a result of millions of years of evolution. There are *countless* nutrients and substances in food that lead to thousands of metabolic reactions when they are consumed. As T. Colin Campbell, PhD, describes it, when it comes to nutrition, the whole is greater than the sum of the individual parts. The nutrients in whole food work together much like a symphony; extract and consume those nutrients apart from the whole, and all bets are off as to their effects.

The complex, harmonious relationship between our bodies and the whole food we eat might explain why the hardworking supplement industry has not been able to produce beneficial products, despite decades of effort and billions of dollars. Consequently, we do not recommend our patients take supplements—with the notable and important exception of vitamin B$_{12}$—unless a specific deficiency arises that cannot be corrected with whole, plant-based foods. Putting aside the bluster of consumer marketing, the research on multivitamin supplements is consistent: They do not demonstrate benefit and may cause harm.[27] A review of twenty-four randomized controlled trials showed "no consistent evidence that the included [vitamin and mineral] supplements affected CVD [cardiovascular disease], cancer, or all-cause mortality in healthy individuals."[28] Single-vitamin supplements have shown similar negative results. In fact, the harm caused by some of them is dramatic. For example, vitamin A, beta-carotene, and vitamin E—while all healthy when consumed in food—have been shown to significantly increase death when consumed as supplements.[29]

The problems with supplements shouldn't come as a surprise. The fact that we need a particular nutrient doesn't mean we need a megadose of it, nor should we consume it in isolation from all the other nutrients and substances it's designed to work with. It may run counter to what we've been taught, but when we think about nutrition, we should think about getting the *right amount* of nutrients; this means obtaining neither too little *nor* too much of them—and being sure they are packaged in the right proportions. Imagine a symphony where we added two hundred extra violins "just to be safe." That would likely sound funny and actually do more harm to the performance than good. It may sound like a difficult task, but in fact it's a most simple one. Like every other species, we should follow nature's lead and simply consume the foods in their natural packaging, which has the perfect amount and balance of nutrients we need.

Given the concerns arising from supplementation, we urge you to resist the latest fads and focus on whole plant foods as your "multivitamin" source. If someone is extolling the virtues of a miracle nutrient pill, you need to be suspicious. The burden of proof should be on them to provide all the information necessary to prove that taking a supplement is going to be more beneficial than not taking it. We should not think for a moment that we are "playing it safe" by taking supplements; the only true way to play it safe is to *not* take those supplements—and to look instead to whole, plant-based foods for the nutrition we need.

Vitamin B$_{12}$

The one exception to the supplement rule is vitamin B$_{12}$, which is important for the development and protection of nerve cells and red blood cells and helps in the production of DNA. Insufficient B$_{12}$ can lead to many health issues, including weakness, fatigue, difficulty concentrating, increased irritability, gastrointestinal distress, anemia, and nervous system dysfunction. B$_{12}$ is the one nutrient that cannot be obtained sufficiently from today's plant-based diet. This is not because we need to eat animal products to obtain it. In fact, animal products themselves don't always contain enough B$_{12}$.[30] The reason for this is that *neither plants nor animals naturally synthesize B$_{12}$*. It is made from bacteria. Animals consume dirt, which is full of bacteria, through the unwashed plants and non-chlorinated water they consume. B$_{12}$ accumulates in the animals' tissues, which becomes a source of the vitamin for humans when we eat the animal.

We humans, on the other hand, rarely eat anything unwashed. In our quest to be clean, we remove the dirt that contains B$_{12}$-producing bacteria from our foods. This sanitary approach certainly has its benefits, as it has decreased our exposure to parasites and other pathogens. As a result, we believe that when you eat a whole-food, plant-based diet, taking a B$_{12}$ supplement is the best way to ensure adequate amounts of the nutrient. There is enough research about supplementing B$_{12}$ that, when taken appropriately, we trust it is beneficial.

VITAMIN D AND THE NEED FOR SUNLIGHT

In contrast to vitamin B$_{12}$, vitamin D is not a nutrient; it's a hormone our body produces when our skin is exposed to the sun's ultraviolet rays. It is very important to have adequate amounts of vitamin D, which is necessary for good health. In fact, low levels of vitamin D are associated with increased rates of cancer, heart disease, and even mortality.[31] Unlike vitamin B$_{12}$, however, vitamin D can and should be obtained through natural sources, namely through exposure to the sun. Sunlight is not only valuable for our vitamin D requirements, but it also improves cognitive function as well as helps in the treatment of various mood disorders, including seasonal affective disorder and clinical depression.[32] So get outside!

Specifically, we recommend that you get out in the sun at least three or four days a week for approximately 5 to 15 minutes depending on your skin type and the UV index; expose as much skin as you can—ideally your face, arms, legs, and even torso, if possible; and make sure you go out when the UV index is 3 or greater (to check your local UV index on any given day, go to www.epa.gov). Just be careful not to burn, as that will *increase* risk of health problems related to sun exposure. We realize that certain work environments as well as geographical limitations—living in areas with a low UV index—can make it difficult to get adequate sun exposure. If these are your circumstances, you should check your vitamin D levels. If you have a vitamin D deficiency (levels less than 20ng/mL), consider two options: UVB light through tanning booths* and/or a supplement.

The reason we strongly recommend sun exposure before supplements is that while vitamin D supplementation will increase your blood levels of the nutrient, it is not clear that this is sufficient to reap the benefits of sunlight exposure. Despite the risks of sun *over*exposure and skin cancer, evidence has shown that *some* sun is beneficial. In fact, in one study, people who worked both indoors and outdoors had less skin cancer than those who worked just indoors or just outdoors.[33] Many randomized studies have confirmed that only in very limited cases (patients with rickets, elderly institutionalized women, etc.) has supplementing with vitamin D pills improved actual health outcomes. And even this benefit has been called into question.[34] Furthermore, vitamin D supplements have associated risks—for example, they have been associated

---

* Tanning booths are more similar to sunlight as far as how we normally produce vitamin D, but caution is recommended. If using a tanning booth, be sure that it does not emit only UVA light, as this will not raise vitamin D levels despite its ability to tan the skin. Also, since the UV index in a tanning booth is high (8 to 10 in an average tanning booth), be careful to avoid overexposure and the resulting skin damage.

with an increased risk of kidney stones.[35] This is not a risk when we get our vitamin D from the sun.

We make these recommendations because it is our best guess that for people who have vitamin insufficiency or deficiency and are unable to obtain adequate sunlight exposure, the benefits of UVB light exposure through certain types of tanning booths—and as a next best option, supplementation—will outweigh the risks of low vitamin D levels. Remember that both tanning booths and supplementation are far less ideal than natural sunlight exposure, so only use them if it is truly necessary. Also, it is important to note that we are talking about small, adequate amounts of sunlight and/or UVB exposure. It is essential that you avoid overexposure and burning of your skin, as that adds significant risk. (The amount of exposure that is adequate for you depends on the UV index and your skin type.)

EXERCISE

Regular exercise is certainly an important part of a healthy lifestyle. Among other things, it's important for bone health, cardiovascular health, and enhancing your sense of well-being. If you're not already exercising, we recommend you find something to get you moving. It's good to do activities you enjoy, which will help you stick to a program. If you can, find activities that are dynamic enough to cover strength, endurance, balance, and flexibility, as all these areas have different benefits on long-term functionality. If your time is severely limited or you are unable to undertake a dynamic program, it's still always better to get out and do *some* activity—even if it's just a short walk each day.

In any case, don't let your inability or unwillingness to exercise prevent you from starting your new eating program. You may be surprised to find that you will still enjoy significant health benefits if you only change the way you eat. But we're happy to report that one of the more wonderful consequences of a whole-food, plant-based diet is that many people gain so much energy they begin to *want* to exercise. Indeed, we've met many friends and read many testimonials from people who were previously sedentary and are now hiking, bicycling, and even competing in athletic events.

If you're already engaged in regular exercise or are a serious athlete, you should *expect* better performance on your new regimen. A whole-food, plant-based diet improves the cardiovascular system, which means better blood flow to the muscles and therefore more efficient delivery of nutrients—all of which translates to more rapid recovery and better physical performance.

IDENTIFY YOUR PERSONAL NEEDS AND PLAN FOR SUCCESS

We *all* have needs, and the ability to recognize and honor them allows us to have greater success in life in general, and in diet and lifestyle change in particular. We identify four primary personal needs below. Review each and consider how you would order them from most to least important to you:

- **Health:** You need to prevent and perhaps reverse disease while improving your quality of life.

- **Pleasure:** You need your food to taste good and you need to feel good.

- **Ease:** You need living this way to be relatively convenient and easy.

- **Acceptance:** You need to be accepted by your friends, family, and coworkers and colleagues, even if your lifestyles are quite different.

After you've identified the order of your needs, reflect on how you will meet each one. Don't worry if you can't say exactly how at this moment. Remember, you're reading this book because you've already determined that you want to make some big lifestyle changes. But the lifestyle you're looking to change has probably been meeting at least *some* of your needs for a while now. For instance, you probably find your current diet reasonably easy to prepare and eat. You likely get pleasure from it, as well as acceptance from your friends, family, and colleagues. It may not, however, be meeting your need for good health—and this is critically important!

The beauty of the Forks Over Knives lifestyle, on the other hand, is that *all* of your needs can be met simultaneously—even while making the changes you desire. A healthy lifestyle, after all, should not alienate loved ones, or be about flavorless foods that take hours to prepare. We will share with you the tools to make it healthy, easy, pleasurable, and acceptable to your family and friends . . . and you will have room to adjust your plan depending on your need at a given moment.

So how does this look in practice? Perhaps right now ease is most important to you, and perhaps you've come to this book ready to jump into your transition 100 percent. This is great, but if you charge ahead and in just a few weeks your need for ease is not being met, you must take the time to consider how you will remedy this. If you don't, you might come to regard perfectly manageable struggles as impossible to overcome and—worse—you might give up.

Your need for ease may be challenged because you're having a hard time finding the right foods, as it is now more difficult to navigate the grocery store than you thought it would be. Or perhaps it's proving to be quite tough to cook in a new way, maybe because you don't have the time to cook or you haven't yet built up a repertoire of dependable and delicious recipes. Acknowledge the issues you're having and seek out achievable solutions. For instance, look for recipes that do not require a lot of preparation. Buy produce that is already chopped and ready for cooking, or rely more on healthy, no-oil-added prepared foods. Prepare foods in bulk and give yourself the time you're going to need to learn new pathways in your grocery store. In other words, try to take a solution-focused approach rather than a problem-focused approach to your new diet and lifestyle. When you run up against an obstacle, focus on how to get around it rather than dwelling on the obstacle itself. This is exactly what we will be helping you with in this book.

There are going to be challenges, but by acknowledging what's important to you and being mindful of when and how your needs aren't being met, you will immeasurably improve your chance for success in both the short and long term. When you take a look at the testimonials in this book, you'll see that many people have enjoyed the success that comes from persevering.

RECOGNIZE YOUR PERSONAL PACE

Just as we all have different primary needs, we also have our own preferred pace in life. Some of us are comfortable moving at a "fast and furious" speed, while others are more "slow and steady." This is a four-week plan because that is usually the time it takes for our patients to get into a real groove—and to begin to reap the benefits of the change. You'll see that in the plan, we change one daily meal per week for the first three weeks—breakfast in Week One, lunch in Week Two, and dinner in Week Three—and we spend the fourth week reflecting on what has worked and what needs further attention as you fine-tune your lifestyle to ensure long-term success. However, you may feel that this pace is too fast or too slow. Feel free to mix it up until you find a pace and methodology that works better for you. For example, you might change breakfast, then wait two weeks before changing lunch. Or you might change a whole day's worth of meals, and do it for just a few days each week until you get the hang of it. Or, after changing breakfast for a few days, you may want to jump all the way in. Use this book in whatever way works best for you. It doesn't matter if you follow the transition schedule exactly as we present it. Everything in this book will still guide you on your path to improved health and wellness. The most important thing is simply that you begin—*now*!

THE LAST WORD: GIVE IT TIME

You've probably been eating a certain way for so long that you know what foods you like and don't like and what works and what doesn't. As you launch your transition, be patient and know that it will take some time to find your way. Your new lifestyle is, well, new! In time, you will figure out what foods and meals you like, and you'll learn how to work around the foods you don't. There is no one food that you *have* to eat. For instance, you may detest black beans or kale—that's fine. We are confident that the knowledge you'll gain from this book will help you discover a whole new repertoire of foods you love. You're *supposed* to enjoy your food. Four weeks from now, you'll *still* enjoy your food—it's just that you'll be enjoying different food than what you eat now.

Above all, keep the big picture in mind. Relax and have fun with your new lifestyle. You're going to be fine. And please don't assess the plan until you've completed all four weeks of the transition. You can't know if it's for you or not until you do. We sometimes see people in the early days stumble a bit and instantly blame their diet change. If you get a headache or are hungry or just don't feel well, it may certainly be something that you ate, but it is *not* a sign that the entire diet is a failure. People endure all sorts of side effects, such as headaches, nausea, and diarrhea, when taking pills that have only *marginal* benefits. This diet, on the other hand, has benefits beyond any pill ever created, so even if a headache or hunger pang develops, please don't let it cause you to run back into the arms of the Standard American Diet. Tweak the Forks Over Knives diet—don't abandon it. The only way to fail is to stop trying.

GETTING PERSONAL

Absolutely everything changed; weight loss, optimal blood pressure and cholesterol, etc. It is difficult to explain how *good* I feel. . . . My husband, Patrick, has been taken off all his heart meds except for one blood pressure pill, after two "mild" heart attacks and the placement of two stents in 2008. A recent follow-up ultrasound shows no heart damage and optimal heart function. . . . I always warn Patrick to beware if I serve him a steak with blue cheese, buttered garlic bread, sour cream–topped potatoes, and Caesar salad—it would be a perfect, unsolvable murder.

—Elizabeth Greenaway, 70, retired, Picton, Ontario, Canada

Achy and inflamed joints limiting my range of motion, sleepless nights, high cholesterol, and feeling chronically tired and exhausted after work (which would prevent me from exercising)—I had thought that this is what getting older is all about . . . aches and pains and depleted energy. I now know otherwise. At first it appeared challenging regarding meal planning. . . . I thought it was going to be more labor intensive and difficult having healthy food on hand, but I viewed it as a new journey and became a health foodie. I purged every animal product from the house immediately after my doctor's recommendation and it really made the transition easier than I thought it would be.

—Leslie Brennecke, 52, teacher, Turlock, CA

Since adopting this lifestyle, I have stopped taking *all* prescription drugs! My aches and pains associated with fibromyalgia have been almost completely diminished. I have so much more energy and vitality than ever before! I sleep great as well. I feel like I finally have control of my life again. I actually feel younger at thirty-five than I did at twenty-five! I have always loved to cook, but now I focus on making delicious recipes that are also healthy.

—Andrea Frasier, 35, Reiki master teacher and transformational coach, Manchester, CT

There is no more counting calories or measuring servings, etc. . . . It's either yes I eat that or no I don't, period. There is no guessing or extensive thinking involved. I no longer feel like I am on a "diet." This is my way of life and it is extremely satisfying and easy to do!

—Claudia Robison, 40, pharmacist, Albuquerque, NM

My motivation has been basically knowing how crazy I was about and in regard to food and the power it held over my life before, and how that insanity is gone now. I look forward to eating now and there's no bargaining, shame, or guilt involved when I sit down to eat. I just eat now—it's been a life changer.

—Stacey Whiteley, 44, program manager, Albany, NY

I don't notice that "click" in my brain anymore that would drive me to one of my former fast-food friends like McDonald's, Burger King, KFC, Popeye's, Wendy's, steakhouses, and BBQ joints. There's been a break in my addiction for sure.

—David Honoré, 46, baker, Chicago, IL

My doctor saw me about six months after I started eating plant strong and stopped in the doorway and asked me "What have you done?" I came prepared with *Forks Over Knives* and *Prevent and Reverse Heart Disease*. Six months later I saw him again and he looked like a new person. I asked him what he had done. He has made the change and now shares the message with his patients.

—Carol Covic, 60, homemaker, Cordova, TN, and Decatur, GA

PART II

WELCOME TO YOUR FOUR-WEEK TRANSITION

I feel in control of my food, not the other way around. I eat what I want to eat and feel good before, during, and after. No more bingeing and regret. In addition to losing forty-five pounds, my blood numbers are now outstanding. Also, I have brought my own lunch to work almost every day for the past two years. I am sure I have saved thousands of dollars.

—Morgan Ewing, 48, retail manager, Westport, CT

For as long as I can remember, following a meal I have always had a sluggish feeling. I have not had that feeling in nearly two years.

—Mark McCloskey, 56, cardiovascular perfusionist, Bellbrook, OH

The easiest thing I found about making the change was once I noticed a difference in the way I felt, it was an easy choice. I felt better both on and off the ice. . . . What a wonderful thing!

—Nick Anderson, 34, professional ice hockey player, Hermantown, MN

Now that we have discussed the benefits of adopting a whole-food, plant-based lifestyle, we hope you're excited and ready to jump right in. What follows is a comprehensive four-week guide that will walk you through each phase of the transition. In each of the next three weeks you will change one meal to plant-based; you'll change breakfast during Week One, lunch during Week Two, and dinner during Week Three. You will spend the final week assessing what is working and fine-tuning anything that needs attention.

In addition to advising you on how to switch each of the three main meals of the day, each week we will discuss—in three recurring features—the most common considerations that are likely to arise:

- **Let's Get Practical** addresses the practical matters that typically come up when people transition to a whole-food, plant-based diet.

- **Eye on Nutrition** deals with the most common nutritional concerns.

- **Making It Work for You** tackles the emotional and psychological challenges that we face as we transition and how to handle them.

Years of patient-care experience have taught us that most questions and concerns come up on a remarkably consistent timetable from patient to patient, so we introduce these considerations largely in the order in which they tend to appear, as follows:

Week One: Change your breakfast

- **Let's Get Practical:** How to read food labels; cleaning out and restocking your pantry and kitchen; going grocery shopping

- **Eye on Nutrition:** Protein

- **Making It Work for You:** Making the mental switch from "diet" to "lifestyle change"

Week Two: Change your lunch

- **Let's Get Practical:** Meal planning and keeping a "food and mood" journal (see page 81)

- **Eye on Nutrition:** Calcium and dairy

- **Making It Work for You:** Food addiction and the myth of willpower

Week Three: Change your dinner

- **Let's Get Practical:** Cooking tips

- **Eye on Nutrition:** Fats

- **Making It Work for You:** Cravings and deprivation

Week Four: Fine-tuning and feeling the freedom of *just eating*

- **Let's Get Practical:** Eating out in restaurants, in others' homes, and while traveling

- **Eye on Nutrition:** Carbohydrates

- **Making It Work for You:** Dealing with social pressures

You'll see throughout the book that we share the inspiring words of people *other* than us who have transitioned into this lifestyle, and whose experiences may help you along the way.

Finally, lest you be concerned that you won't know how to begin to prepare your first meal, we have included nearly one hundred delicious recipes at the end of the book. Here you will find everything from the simplest dip, smoothie, and wrap to delectable soups, casseroles, and pasta dishes. We want to make sure that you have what you need to plan every aspect of your next four weeks, and beyond!

I eat more now than before. No calorie-counting or silly watching over what I eat. No denial. I embrace the bountiful plant-based whole foods I can eat, and it's endless.

—Juliette Arnold, 49, self-employed, Montara, CA

My husband and I started looking at grocery stores in a whole new way. The marketing and sales ploys disgusted us and we are now able to spend minimal time among the prepackaged, processed aisles and get back to Mother Nature at her best.

—Laura Galvin, 45, wood mill worker, Birchwood, WI

I allowed myself to indulge in more exotic fruits and veggies since a budget without expensive meats and cheeses gave me more flexibility.

—Ulli Nelson, 50, registered nurse, Elgin, TX

WEEK ONE: **The Forks Over Knives Breakfast**

Now that you're ready to get started, begin your transition with the very first meal of the week. In Week One, you'll restructure your breakfast so that you start every day with a whole-food, plant-based meal. We'll also talk about how to read food labels, clean out and restock your pantry, tell you what you need to know about protein, and help you make the mental switch from merely dieting to changing your lifestyle.

The most important first step this week (and every other week) is to make a plan. In Week Two, we'll delve deeper into developing a successful meal plan strategy. This week your task is simple: Write down what you plan to have for breakfast every day. To help you decide what your plan should look like, think about what your typical breakfast looks like—it's helpful to jot down what you ate for breakfast the last week or two. Now, create a whole-food, plant-based breakfast blueprint for the week that has just as much or as little diversity. If you are a creature of habit, you may be happy to eat the same bowl of oatmeal each and every morning. If you prefer a little day-to-day variety, you may want to have that oatmeal one morning, steel-cut oats the next, and oil-free granola on another day. Or for lots of variation, try oats one day, a smoothie with a bowl of fruit the next, a breakfast wrap on another, pancakes another day, and a large bowlful of clementines on another. (See pages 141–153 for a selection of breakfast recipes, and the Resources on page 299 for great books and online sources for recipes.) Whatever your choice of food, make sure you plan to—and do—eat *enough*.

Even though you're embarking on a new lifestyle, don't forget to keep eating the whole, plant-based foods you already love. Sometimes you might want to keep it really simple and eat as much as you can of a single favorite food for a meal. For example, if grains are your thing, try two or more big bowls of quinoa or cracked wheat. For our part, we love fruit and sometimes make a breakfast of as much melon as we can eat. Yes, fruit by itself makes a great meal. If you think "fruit for breakfast" means grabbing a banana or an apple as you run out the door, you need to radically expand this definition for your new lifestyle. You need to be sure to eat a sufficient volume to make a meal. A Forks Over Knives fruit breakfast can be half (or even all!) a watermelon or a pint of raspberries and several bananas. And that bowl of clementines we just mentioned may hold a dozen or more whole fruits!

It is important not to "drink" your calories or food whenever possible, especially if you are trying to lose weight or reverse certain diseases like diabetes.[36] Liquid calories lack sufficient bulk to fill you up. We think a little plant milk or juice is fine on cereal or to flavor foods when cooking. However, we recommend that you avoid drinking glasses of extracted juices, plant milks, sodas, energy drinks, and other sweetened beverages. Smoothies, unlike juices, contain all parts of the food, although they still provide less bulk due to the blending process. As such, smoothies can be enjoyed occasionally, if desired, but should not be a major part of the diet.

You may have heard that you have to eat a variety of foods at a given meal. This is a myth. If you are interested in variety, it can easily be achieved over time; however, simplicity at the meal provides many practical benefits and is perfectly okay—plus it can be very enjoyable. Focus on whole food and eat the foods that you love—it's that simple.

As you go through this first week, think of your plan as your guide, not your albatross. If you find that a dish you've eaten one morning doesn't really satisfy you—perhaps you're hungry for lunch an hour earlier than usual or you don't feel as good as usual—do not assume that the entire Forks Over Knives lifestyle is not for you. Instead, tweak the rest of the meal plan this week to address whatever isn't working. If you are getting hungrier sooner than you would like, then either increase the volume or calorie density (see page 34) of breakfast the next day—for example, instead of a single bowl of oatmeal piled with fruit, have *two* full bowls of oatmeal with the same total amount of fruit—or add an additional snack afterward. You can play around with this as needed to fit your lifestyle. Once you have created your meal plan, write up your shopping list for the full week. This way you can buy everything you'll need for the week's breakfasts during a single trip to the grocery store (see pages 65–67).

The important thing to keep in mind this week is that you must eat until you feel comfortably satisfied. Give yourself the time you need to reach this point, even if it means setting your alarm clock to wake you fifteen minutes earlier.

LET'S GET PRACTICAL

How to Read Nutrition Labels: A Checklist

One of the most critical things we teach our patients is actually among the easiest for you to teach yourself: how to decipher labels. We don't like to focus too much on this because we want you to primarily eat whole, unprocessed foods, and these foods don't generally have labels. (Or if they do—on a bag of lentils or a can of beans, for instance—they're straightforward enough not to require deciphering.) But we live in the same world that you do, and we know that some packaged foods are likely to become or remain staples in your pantry. Oil-free condiments, plant-based milks, whole cereals and granolas, and chips and crackers are some of the minimally processed and packaged items that are in our kitchen right now, and they'll likely be in yours, too. So let's review what to look for on these labels:

1 **Check the ingredients.** Ideally, there will be very few total ingredients. We hesitate to give a hard and fast number because some products we buy—condiments or muesli, for example—have more individual ingredients than we'd be comfortable with in chips or crackers.

If you're buying a grain product, **make sure it contains whole (not refined) grains.** Whole grains contain the entire grain kernel—the bran, germ, and endosperm. Look for these ingredients at the top of the ingredient list: brown rice, buckwheat, bulgur, millet, oatmeal, quinoa, rolled oats, whole-grain barley, whole-grain corn, whole-grain sorghum, whole-grain triticale, whole oats, whole rye, whole wheat, and wild rice. The terms *multigrain, stone-ground, 100 percent wheat, cracked wheat, seven-grain, durum,* or *bran* may sound good, but they do not indicate that the ingredient is a whole grain.[37]

2 **Check the serving size.** Look closely at the serving size and total number of servings in the package. Some companies make the product appear healthier than it is by reporting information on an unrealistically small serving size. Many cans of soup, for instance, could reasonably serve one person, but they are considered two or more servings, so the information on the nutrition label looks better. Another egregious example of serving size deception are those of spray oils, which consider a serving size to be so small that their labels actually say they have *no* fat per serving, when in fact they are almost 100 percent fat. With small enough serving sizes, amounts of fat, sodium, and other unhealthy components can seem much smaller than they are.

3 **Check the fat.** You should aim for foods with less than 15 percent of cal-ories from fat, which allows for only a minimal amount of your food to contain a higher percentage than that. (Note that it is fine if you're over 15 percent at a single meal; it's *over time* that you should average less than 15 percent.)

To figure out what percentage of calories comes from fat, divide the calories from fat by the total calories per serving—both are listed on the same line of the "nutrition facts" label—and multiply the result by 100.

Calculating Percentage of Calories from Fat

Nutrition Facts
Serving Size 2 Tortillas (48g)
Serving Per Container 6

Amount Per Serving

Calories 120   Calories from Fat 15

% Daily Value*

Total Fat 2g	**3%**
Saturated Fat 0g	**0%**
Trans Fat 0g	**0%**
Cholesterol 0mg	**0%**
Sodium 10mg	**0%**
Total Carbohydrate 23g	**8%**
Dietary Fiber 3g	**13%**
Sugars 1g	
Protein 3g	

To calculate the percentage of calories that come from fat, divide the calories from fat by total calories and multiply by 100:

$$(15 \div 120) \times 100 = 12.5 \text{ percent}$$

4 **Check the sodium.** Aim to keep the sodium no higher than 1 mg per calo-rie, unless the product is a condiment or you're using just a small amount of it as part of a larger recipe. So, for example, a food that is 100 calories per serving should have no more than 100 mg of sodium per serving.

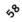

5 **Check the added sugar.** Ingredients are listed on labels in descending order by weight, which means that a product contains more of the first ingredients listed than the last. Avoid any product that includes sugar as one of the first three ingredients (unless there are only three total ingredients listed, and sugar is last). Some companies profit from the weight rule on the label and hide how much added sugar is actually in a product. Instead of adding just one type of sugar, they add two or more, and the total weight of each of these is small enough that they are buried in the list. You want to generally avoid products that use this "multiple listing" trick, keeping in mind that added sugar can come in many forms that don't include the word *sugar*. Look for brown rice syrup, cane juice, corn syrup, dextrose, fructose, lactose, sucrose, honey, and molasses, among many others.

Cleaning Out Your Kitchen and Pantry

Now that you understand how to read nutrition labels, it's time to take a good look at the food that's in your house right now and clean out the refrigerator, freezer, and pantry. This may sound like a daunting and even wasteful exercise, but we prefer to think of it as a gift you give yourself. We do realize that this week we've only told you how to transition to whole-food, plant-based breakfasts, so if you would prefer to hold on to some of your current supplies for lunch and dinner, that's just fine. That said, the more you can clean out now the better, for getting rid of the less-than-healthy and out-and-out junk foods in your house is one of the most helpful things you can do right now. It means that the next time you're craving something that's not good for you, you'll need to actively leave home to get it. This challenges our innate desire for ease and convenience. You're more likely to just grab something from the refrigerator or pantry rather than run out to the store. By ensuring that you have only healthy options, you transform your kitchen into a satisfying and nourishing oasis, rather than a minefield of processed and high-oil foods.

So roll up your sleeves and start purging! Get rid of any foods that are highly processed; not plant-based; contain oil; or are high in sugar, salt, or fat.

The exceptions to the last category are avocados, nuts, seeds, and natural nut or seed butters. These are higher-fat whole foods that we use sparingly.

Once you've tossed the unhealthy stuff, take a moment to enjoy the extra space. But don't get too used to it, because we have no intention of leaving you with empty shelves! Now you get to create a kitchen pantry that's healthy, exciting, and inspiring. From now on, when you get cravings (and if you're human, it'll happen) you'll have satisfying choices. See below for a list of healthy options for your refrigerator, freezer, and pantry.

When you are more comfortable with the changes you are making, you will see patterns evolve. For instance, you may find you make certain recipes frequently, so you'll want to have the ingredients for those recipes on hand. Or, you may notice that you gravitate toward specific foods as snacks and "craving" indulgences. Make sure they are always in your pantry so that you're less likely to give in to hankerings for unhealthy options.

Now it's time to stock your kitchen the Forks Over Knives way. Below is a list of staples for a well-stocked whole-food, plant-based kitchen and pantry. For optimum health, be sure to buy the oil-free (as well as low-fat and low-sodium when possible and available) versions of these items.

The Well-Stocked Refrigerator

- Fresh salsa—store-bought or homemade (page 274)

- Dips and sauces, such as hummus, baba ghanoush, bean and lentil dips, etc.—store-bought or homemade (see pages 258–274)

- Jelly or jam

- Plant-based milk* (see Note, page 61)

- Fresh fruits, including some cut up for grab-and-go access

- Fresh vegetables, including some cut up for grab-and-go access

- Steamed vegetables, such as green beans, broccoli, snap peas, cauliflower

- Roasted or baked potatoes and/or sweet potatoes

- Cooked grain of the week (page 81)

- Cooked bean of the week (page 81)

- Corn or wheat tortillas

The Well-Stocked Freezer

- Vegetables, such as corn, artichoke hearts, peas, spinach, green beans,
mushrooms, and broccoli

- Fruits, such as blueberries, mangoes, strawberries, and cherries

- Frozen cooked grains such as brown rice and quinoa

- Homemade "TV dinners" (page 81)

The Well-Stocked Fresh Pantry

- Potatoes—all varieties, including white, sweet, purple, etc.

- Onions and/or shallots

- Garlic

- Fresh ginger

- Lemons and limes

The Well-Stocked Pantry

Note: *We use items marked with an asterisk occasionally and sparingly, either as condiments or in small amounts to accompany meals or snacks.*

- Dried beans, such as pinto, black, and kidney

- Canned beans (dried are cheaper, but keep a few cans on hand for quick meals and snacks)—all kinds, including fat-free refried beans

- Grains, such as barley, brown rice, buckwheat, bulgur, millet, quinoa, polenta, rye, wheat berries, and whole wheat couscous

- Canned vegetables (we think fresh or frozen taste better, but it's always good to have a few cans for last-minute meals)—corn, artichokes, and roasted red peppers are especially tasty

- Canned tomatoes (whole, diced, and crushed), including seasoned and fire-roasted

- Plain tomato sauce and tomato paste

- Pasta sauces

- Pasta made from whole wheat, rice, or quinoa or any other whole grain or legume

- Whole-grain pizza crust, such as Kabuli brand

- Plant-based milk, such as rice, oat, almond, or soy, in shelf-stable packaging (refrigerate after opening)★

- Oatmeal—rolled oats and/or steel-cut oats

- Cold cereals

- Dried fruit, such as dates, prunes, and raisins★

- Baked tortilla chips

- Popcorn kernels for air popping

- Rice cakes or corn thins

- Whole-grain rice or wheat crackers

- Bottled salsa

- Dip and dressing mixes, such as those made by Simply Organic★

- Salad dressings★

- Vegetable broth

- Natural sweeteners, such as maple syrup, brown rice syrup, and pure cane sugar (optional)★

- Unsweetened applesauce

- Condiments, such as mustard, ketchup, barbeque sauces, and vegan Worcestershire sauce*

- Vinegars such as rice, white wine, red wine, and cider

- Soy sauce and/or tamari*

- Hot sauce, such as Tabasco*

- Nut butters, such as peanut, almond, and sunflower seed (optional)— choose those with no added oil (after opening and stirring, store in the refrigerator to keep them from separating)*

- Whole wheat pastry flour

- Cornmeal

- Aluminum-free baking powder

- Arrowroot powder

The Well-Stocked Spice and Dried Herb Cabinet

- Basil

- Bay leaves

- Black peppercorns (for pepper grinder) or ground black pepper

- Cayenne pepper and/or chipotle powder

- Chili powder

- Cilantro

- Crushed red pepper

- Curry powder

- Dill

- Garlic powder (not garlic salt)

- Ground cinnamon

- Ground cumin

- Ground ginger

- Italian seasoning

- Marjoram

- Nutmeg (whole berries for grating)

- Onion powder

- Oregano

- Paprika and/or smoked paprika

- Parsley

- Sage

- Salt (sea and/or kosher)

- Turmeric

Shopping Without Breaking a Sweat—or the Bank

A list of unfamiliar foods you can't locate can make the grocery store you've been shopping in for years seem entirely strange and new to you. Grocery shopping can be plenty daunting even when you know exactly what you want and where to find it. If you're like us, the hustle and bustle of other shoppers and long lines is not your idea of a good time—we all have precious little free time as it is.

Rest assured that as with any new experience, **practice makes it easier**. Think of the very first time you traveled to a new job or school. At first, the route was unfamiliar to you, but after several days it became routine, and after several months you perfected not just one way but several ways of getting there. Food shopping is no exception: The more you do it, the more straightforward it becomes. Locating new items may be a headache the first couple of times. Over time, as many of the ingredients you use regularly repeat themselves on your list and you become more comfortable in previously unexplored aisles of your supermarket, your shopping excursions will be more efficient. Eventually a new routine will emerge and become habit.

But before we can get to that practiced ease, we have to make our very first Forks Over Knives meal plan and shopping list. This week you're changing your first meal of the day, so start there: Replace the ingredients you typically buy for a week of your usual breakfasts with the ingredients for an equal number of whole-food, plant-based meals. Begin now to make a habit of the following routines:

First, **build your shopping list at the same time you build your meal plan**. In fact, use the same sheet of paper for your meal plan and the corresponding shopping list for the week. In time you'll have a good collection of these ready-to-go documents, each with a week of meal plans and shopping lists so you can easily alternate among them. We'll talk more about this next week (see page 79).

Second, **schedule your shopping and do some advance preparation**. Decide when you can do your cooking and plan your shopping accordingly. Then you should put "grocery shopping" on your calendar—just as you do for any other appointment. If, for example, you plan to cook Thursday, schedule a stop at the store on Wednesday after work. Or set aside time during the weekend to do both the shopping and some preparation: It won't take much more than an hour to steam a big pot of the grain or the bean of the week (or both) and chop a bunch of vegetables for several days of meals. (It'll take even less time to cook that grain if you have a rice cooker, which we consider a minimal investment that has repaid us many times over in ease and convenience. Similarly, a pressure cooker is a big time-saver for cooking beans, legumes, and other vegetables.) And while you're at it, cut up some fruit and trim and steam or bake some vegetables. Now there will be something ready to eat when you get hungry. This is always important, but especially during the first few weeks, when you are still adjusting to this new way of eating. The more this becomes habit, the easier it will be. We'll talk a bit more about this in Week Three (see page 99).

Third, **focus on what's important and remember what's not**. Too often our patients tell us they don't eat fruits and vegetables because they cannot afford to, but this is because of a misunderstanding of what a whole-food, plant-based diet is. We can't stress enough that the diet is absolutely possible without breaking the bank.

Eating the Forks Over Knives way does not mean you have to buy the priciest foods from the highest-end grocery stores in town. The foundation of this diet is carbohydrate-based whole food, such as potatoes, beans, and rice—all staples that are among the least expensive foods you can buy, no matter where you live.

And while some people prefer to eat only organic, fresh food, from a health perspective this is not absolutely necessary. Most modern diseases that afflict people are not the result of the difference between organic and conventional produce, fresh and frozen broccoli, or canned and dried beans. Whether our diets lead to health or sickness is determined by the significant difference between whole, plant-based foods on the one side and animal-based and highly processed foods on the other. We should not let our need for convenient, affordable food—including shortcuts, such as canned and frozen as well as less expensive conventional produce—deter us from consuming the whole, plant-based foods that will stave off disease.

Finally, **don't overlook how economical it is to buy—and cook—in bulk**. So many plant-based foods lend themselves to longer storage that it's very easy to shop and cook this way. Grains, dried beans and legumes, and even cereals can be bought in bulk at many stores. When stored in airtight containers in dark cabinets, they'll often last for months. Cook a couple of pounds of dried beans or legumes at a time, then freeze them in individual two-cup containers, and you'll have the equivalent of many cans for a fraction of the price. Even cooked grains can be packed in freezer bags and stored—they're delicious stirred into soup after defrosting. Also, while you'll no longer want to hit the dairy and meat cases at warehouse club stores, such as Costco, they do sell plenty of whole, plant-based foods, including large bags of grains and legumes, as well as a variety of canned beans and vegetables in cases of six or twelve, which are usually less expensive than buying them individually.

It is important, especially now, at the beginning of your journey, to keep in mind how many choices you have. A lot of people considering transitioning to a plant-based diet worry they will be relegated to a life of steamed vegetables, brown rice, and salads—so plain and boring it's enough to make many people run to the nearest barbecue joint! But nothing could be further from the truth. The Forks Over Knives lifestyle includes many of the foods you already enjoy: pancakes, lasagna, pizza, risotto, stir-fries, tacos, and so much more. You will even enjoy desserts. Use the "Well-Stocked" lists above and the recipes in this book (beginning on page 137) as your launchpad for finding plenty of bold flavors and easy recipes to make your transition easier than you could have imagined.

EYE ON NUTRITION: PROTEIN

You are not alone if you are asking, "Where will I get my protein?" This is by far the most frequently asked question we hear. (If, instead, you're wondering about calcium—the second most common question from our patients—we discuss it in Week Two, page 77.) Long after you have moved on from this book and fully embraced your whole-food, plant-based lifestyle, we promise that you, too, will be asked where you get your protein.

The truth is that most people, including those who ask you if and how you're getting enough protein, don't really know how much protein our bodies require to be healthy and strong. Furthermore, people believe this single nutrient is so important and difficult to get that we must actively pursue foods that contain high amounts of it, even when those foods compromise our health. The overall "package" of nutrients in meat, fish, poultry, dairy, and eggs is harmful and makes us vulnerable to chronic diseases. The notion that we must make ourselves sick to get enough protein is woefully misconceived.

Let's get to some answers, beginning with a quick review of the basics: Protein, carbohydrates, and fat are the three primary macronutrients our bodies can use for energy. Twenty individual amino acids are the building blocks for protein and are fundamental to a great number of vital functions in your body, everything from building and repairing cells to creating antibodies and enzymes. You can actually synthesize most of these amino acids on your own. The eight that the adult body cannot produce are called the *essential* amino acids because you must get them from your food. (Children need a ninth amino acid, also easily obtained through plant foods, but our bodies develop the ability to synthesize this one when we reach adulthood.)

If it is so easy to meet your protein requirements with a whole-food, plant-based diet, then why do people worry about getting enough? It is likely because we have been led to believe that primarily animal-based foods contain sufficient protein and, furthermore, that we *need* to eat those foods to avoid becoming protein deficient. The reality is that protein deficiency is almost exclusively seen in people suffering from a *calorie* deficiency. In these cases, there will be an overall nutrient deficiency, not just a protein deficiency, and when this happens the concern should be getting more calories and all nutrients—not just more protein.

As for how much protein you need, the answer is the amount that a diet of whole, plant-based foods provides you. All whole, plant-based foods have protein. We know from our extensive review of the research and our experience in our practice that people thrive on a plant-based diet without ever going out of their way to find "sources" of protein. Indeed, it's not a mystery that we've evolved over millions of years without ever aiming for a "source" of this or any other nutrient. Yet the mistaken notion that we need to go out of our way to consume certain individual nutrients is pervasive, and protein is the nutrient most commonly identified as one you must target to ensure you get enough. But we're not interested in trying to achieve arbitrary targets; we're interested in achieving good health. And the best way to achieve good health is by targeting whole plant foods, not numbers of grams of protein.

When you eat a diet based on fruit, vegetables, tubers, whole grains, and legumes about 10 percent of your total calorie intake will be from protein. To see this in action, take a look at a few of our recipes: The Quickest Breakfast Wrap (page 145) clocks in at about 10.3 percent protein, the Spinach-Potato Tacos (page 170) are around 12.1 percent, the Shepherd's Pot Pie (page 224) hits 11.6 percent, the Lentil-Vegetable Stew (page 194) is 23.0 percent, and even the Chewy Lemon-Oatmeal Cookies (page 278) are 9.3 percent protein.[38] We list these percentages only to demonstrate how common plant-based foods contain sufficient amounts of this nutrient—not as any kind of guide to choosing what whole, plant-based foods to eat. In fact, you should not worry about how much protein you're getting any more than you should worry about the perfect number of breaths you take in a day. Nevertheless, if you're still worried that 10 percent isn't adequate, in a moment we'll discuss the very real dangers of consuming *too much* protein—especially when it comes from animal sources.

The **Incomplete** Protein Myth

Experts once believed that we could not get our essential amino acids from plants. Researchers inched a little closer to the truth when they discovered that we can get protein from plants but faltered in arbitrarily categorizing "complete" and "incomplete" proteins, the only difference being that the *concentration* of amino acids per gram of an "incomplete" protein source is less than that of a "complete" protein source. In disseminating this myth, they encouraged food combining of "incomplete" proteins in order to get a "complete" protein (i.e., eating beans and rice). Contrary to popular belief, however, "incomplete" proteins contain all of the same eight essential amino acids that are found in "complete" proteins. Unfortunately, this definition does little to benefit and a lot to harm our health these days by guiding us toward animal foods over plant foods as our preferred source of protein, when, in fact, a diet solely of plants easily meets our needs for all eight essential amino acids, *without* food pairing and combining. The bottom line is this: virtually every plant food has all eight of the essential amino acids; it's only the *concentrations* of some of the amino acids that differ. However, even though the amino acids may be present in lower concentrations, these foods are in no way lacking.

The Dangers of Protein Overconsumption

We have never once in our practice seen a single patient suffering from protein deficiency. On the other hand, we treat many, many people suffering from heart disease, diabetes, and other chronic diseases that result directly from striving to get lots of protein. We know for certain that more is *not* better.

Many Americans consume up to 35 percent or more of their calories from protein, which is *much* more than twice as much as they need. That may not strike you as a particularly big deal. You may wonder, what's the problem with eating more protein than we need? It's not like we're talking about sugar or fat. We *know* those are bad. But protein is good!

Actually, overconsumption of protein is a *very* big deal. When we consume more than we need, we don't just pee out the surplus as we do some other nutrients. Remember your high school chemistry class where you learned that acids and bases neutralize each other? Our bodies are more basic (alkaline) and they prefer to stay that way. As we've already discussed, protein is made up of amino *acids*, and as such it is acidic by nature. Animal products aren't simply high in all proteins; they are particularly elevated in those amino acids that are more highly sulfuric and acidic. Breaking these down taxes our bodies, and when we consume too much of this sort of protein it stresses our kidneys, liver, and bones, among other things. Too much protein can lead to kidney stress or damage, kidney stones, calcium loss, and osteoporosis.[39] A recent study even found that a diet high in animal protein can lead to an earlier death compared to a diet with less animal protein.[40]

T. Colin Campbell, PhD, has demonstrated both in lab studies and in population studies in rural China—and written about extensively (most notably in his book *The China Study*, coauthored with his son Thomas M. Campbell, MD)— that consuming high amounts of protein from animal sources is associated not only with higher individual instances of diseases, such as cancer and cardiovascular disease, but also with faster-growing cancer cells and more aggressive disease. In his laboratory work, Dr. Campbell found that higher amounts of protein from plant sources, on the other hand, did not promote cancer.

What About Athletes?

Do athletes protein-load before a big event? No, they *carb* load! This is because the body's preferred fuel is carbohydrates, required to replenish glycogen, the form in which carbs are stored in our bodies. When carbs are not replenished or when we consume high-protein diets, we can encounter fatigue, decreased endurance, fluid loss, and possible dehydration.[41] In fact, in pursuing animal-based foods for protein, you'll be driving up the percentage of dietary protein, and frequently driving down the percentage of carbohydrates. You'll be getting more protein calories that you *don't* need at the expense of carbohydrate calories that you *do* need—for fuel.

Athletes do require more protein (and all nutrients) than sedentary people, but there is no evidence that they require a *higher percentage* of protein compared to other macronutrients in their diet to perform more optimally. To put it another way, a diet with 10 percent protein is sufficient for most people, athlete and nonathlete alike. If an average adult female eats 2,000 calories, 10 percent is 200 calories from protein. If an average female *athlete* eats 3,000 calories, 10 percent is 300 calories from protein—that's a 50 percent increase in protein achieved by simply eating more of the same foods. So when you exercise, you don't need to change the composition of the food (i.e., consuming foods with higher concentrations of protein or consuming protein powders). You just need to eat more of the same foods. The increased athletic activity will work up your hunger drive. In response, you will consume more protein as well as nutrients of all types. This works well since physical activity likely requires more of all nutrients, not just protein.

The beauty is that nature has figured it out. We move more, we eat more. All we have to do is eat whole, plant-based foods, which have ratios of protein and carbs and all other nutrients in the proper proportions.

The Takeaway: Protein

Protein is essential for proper body functioning. Since there's more than enough protein on a whole-food, plant-based diet, you should focus on the foods you enjoy and not worry about targeting specific foods to meet an arbitrary requirement. The bottom line on protein is simple: just eat!

MAKING IT WORK FOR YOU

Making the Mental Switch from "Diet" to "Lifestyle"

At the beginning of the book we talked about how fraught the word *diet* is in America and how it brings to mind unpleasant words (and feelings), like *deprivation* and *portion control.* Diets tend to emphasize what we should *not* eat rather than all the delicious things we *can* enjoy. Diets compel us to fixate on restriction and portion sizes, leaving us feeling hungry and miserable. And worst of all, diets rely on "willpower," that elusive virtue that will almost always crumble, right along with our self-confidence.

Dieting guides and gurus tend to make the point that no matter how tasty something on their plan might be, portion control is a key to success. The unfortunate irony, though, is that portion control is actually one of the primary reasons for *failure* on standard diets. This is because portion control and restriction lead to deprivation, which is not a feeling we can live with for too long (we'll talk more about this on page 91). We strongly recommend that you stop thinking about portion control entirely by thinking of this as a lifestyle not a diet. From now on, we recommend you eat until you are comfortably satisfied, even if that means you're eating considerably more volume in a single sitting than you're accustomed to. This isn't an empty promise. It's science. As you'll recall, whole, plant-based foods have lower calorie density (page 34) than animal products and processed foods, which means that you will need to eat larger, *not* smaller, portions.

In these early days you must listen to your body not only during meals, but afterward. If you're hungry sooner than usual after a meal, it probably means you need to eat more. You must give yourself the time to figure out how to react to familiar feelings in new ways. Make sure you have a well-stocked kitchen so that when you're tempted to fall into the old habits you employed to stave off hunger or cravings, you instead have a selection of healthy, whole foods to turn to. (Refer to the lists on pages 59–65 to help stock your pantry and fridge.)

Now is a good time to reread pages 40–43 in chapter 3 and revisit the personal needs you identified for yourself at the start. It's very important to recognize that you will always have these needs. Periodically refocusing your efforts on what is most important to you—ease, pleasure, health, or acceptance—as well as what strategies can help meet *all* of those needs is a great plan for success.

Finally, keep in mind that the more realistic you are with yourself along your path, the greater your chance for sustainable results. Choose a pace you believe you can stick to, and be flexible about changing it as necessary. Sure, it's true that big changes lead to big results, but incremental changes count, too. Our goal here is long-term success. It's less desirable to make huge leaps this week if that will lead you to flounder and fail. Commit to the small steps that you can establish gradually and then maintain over the next ten, twenty, or fifty years. Success begets success, and we believe each step forward is likely to bring you increased confidence, motivation, and understanding of how to achieve your goals.

GETTING PERSONAL

We decided to try eating plant-based for one month. At the three-week mark, my husband turned to me and announced that he didn't want to go back to our old way of eating because he felt so good. We found that knowing we could get all our protein requirements from plants made us relax and not worry if we were getting enough protein.

—Anne Barber, 49, self-employed, Winnipeg, Manitoba, Canada

It was so much easier to cook with just a few basic pantry items (canned beans, pasta, rice, canned tomatoes, veggie broth, and spices)—you just need some fresh veggies and you have glorious food to eat in a few easy steps! I have a handful of go-to recipes and I just never get tired of them, they are so delicious. It was also much cheaper—my grocery bill has been reduced by more than half by eliminating meat (including dairy), probably more like 75 percent. Plus, we hardly ever eat out anymore, as everyone (including me) much prefers my cooking to any restaurant.

—Carol-Ann Kiartanson, 50, professional accountant, Winnipeg, Manitoba, Canada

Grocery shopping has become easier than I thought it would be, and after a few new pantry items were in place, grocery bills went down. So that was wonderful.

—Sarah Bjork, 27, administrative assistant, St. Paul, MN

I see this getting easier as restaurants and grocery chains begin to accommodate vegan eaters. We are amazed and encouraged to see Costco's shelves growing with low-fat, whole-grain, vegan options.

—Jon Thrasher, 58, international business consultant, Charlotte, NC

I have rediscovered my love of cooking. Within two to three weeks, I developed recipes such that I eat only food I love at every meal, and I don't have to limit quantities or count anything. I felt better, so it turned out to be easy to keep eating whole-food, plant-based.

—Dan'l Leviton, 56, software architect, Monrovia, CA

The foods I am eating now are far more varied and satisfying than they were before. Previously, they satisfied a fleeting craving, only to cause the malaise of a lunch coma, if not indigestion or worse. The lunch coma is a thing of the past, as are the cravings now that I have broken my body of this unhealthy habit.

—Eric Robertson, 28, computer programmer, software development manager, West Bloomfield, MI

Once I started eating only plant-based foods I had a clear sense that this was what my body needed. When I was tempted at times to have a burger or some other gut-busting delicacy, I would give myself ten or fifteen minutes to think about how it tasted and enjoy the memory. Then I would remember how it used to make my body feel.

—Teresa Ingram, 60, retired accountant, Sacramento, CA

WEEK TWO: **The Forks Over Knives Lunch**

CHAPTER 5

Now you have one week under your belt. Way to go! Don't worry if you're not completely plant-based for breakfast yet or if you're still tweaking your morning meals. You should still move ahead with this week, when you'll switch to whole-food, plant-based lunches. Progressing to the next step in your transition will increase your opportunities to try even more new foods and expand your repertoire. In fact, we think that whenever you're feeling a little stalled, the best option is to keep charging ahead rather than waiting to get everything just right. The more whole, plant-based meals you eat, the more you'll discover foods that you love, and the easier your transition will become. To that end, take a look in your pantry and kitchen and try to get rid of any unhealthy lunch items that you didn't feel ready to part with during your pantry purge last week. We'll give you a little boost this week in our Let's Get Practical section, where we'll delve deeper into meal planning. We also suggest keeping a food and mood journal, a good way to track your progress so that if you are having some issues it'll be easier to figure out what's going on. Plus, we'll turn our Eye on Nutrition to the subject of calcium. Finally, this week, we'll tackle the very real issue of food addiction and the myth of willpower.

Since this is the first time you've planned a full week of whole-food, plant-based lunches, just begin by writing down everything you can remember eating for lunch over the past week or two. Next, create a list with a week of whole-food, plant-based lunches—either by simply modifying what you already typically like to eat for lunch or by trying out entirely new meals. We'll talk more about this a little further on. As you make your lunch meal plan for this week, use whatever you learned last week about how you feel when you eat a full meal of whole, plant-based foods. Were you hungry after breakfast earlier than usual on the first day or two? Go ahead and adjust the volume of what you're eating so that you're satiated until the next meal. Recall what worked and what didn't and apply those lessons to your lunch planning. (Check out the recipes in the back of this book for ideas, as well as the Resources on page 299 for great books and online sources for recipes.)

For lunch, we enjoy all sorts of different foods: Soups and stews, potato or grain dishes, and sandwiches are great options, as are pizza or burritos with all the fixings. And of course anything on the dinner menu can be on the lunch menu, too. Keep in mind what we've talked about with calorie density (see page 30). If you're trying to lose weight, stay on the lower end of the calorie density scale. For example, wrap your sandwich in fresh green leaves like romaine or collards because they have lower calorie density than bread and pita (page 34), or just use one slice of bread instead of two. Another tip if you're trying to lose weight is to "front load"—that is, eat a low-calorie-density dish or food before your meal, such as a piece or several pieces of fruit, a bowl of tossed greens, or a bowl of soup.

If you're usually a soup-and-salad person at lunchtime, there are plenty of both available to you. Remember, though, that eating until you are satiated is vital, so don't assume that a green salad and light, brothy soup will do the trick. Be realistic, and consider hearty soups and salads based on whole grains or beans.

If you eat out at restaurants often, consider the style and menu of the places you ordinarily go. Do you believe they can easily accommodate your plant-based diet? Depending on where you live, your local restaurants may already have offerings that can be customized to your new lifestyle. If vegetable soup is on the menu, have a bowl along with a side of steamed grains or pasta that you can stir in to make the soup more filling. Green salads are offered nearly everywhere, of course, but as mentioned earlier, unless they're large and contain beans and grains, they're unlikely to be filling enough to hold you over until your next meal. And be careful with salads in restaurants; they are often doused in oil-based dressings, which are unhealthy and calorie dense. You're better off asking for a plate of grilled vegetables with grains or a baked potato with an oil-free sauce or condiment. Thinking ahead is the best way to stay on track. (We talk more about eating at restaurants in Week Four (see page 117). Don't forget to maintain your breakfast plan this week as well!

LET'S GET PRACTICAL

Meal Planning

We've already talked a lot about how important it is to make a plan each week. We emphasize this because not only is it a good way to transition to a whole-food, plant-based diet, it's also the best way we know to live this way for a lifetime. No matter what stage you're at, creating a meal plan every week makes life easier. And in the early stages it will keep you accountable to yourself. Create the plan and shopping list in a calm moment and you're much less likely to end up at the grocery store, knowing there's not really anything to eat at home and so overwhelmed by the options that you're suddenly making decisions on the fly. This is when you're more likely to be impulsive and may even fall back into the familiar patterns from before you began your transition. A plan empowers you to remain true to the promise you have made to yourself to choose a lifestyle that will enable both good health *and* satisfaction.

You can certainly continue as you began with breakfast last week: Simply list your planned meals based on what you've eaten for lunch recently and create a separate shopping list. But we prefer a slightly more structured system. We use it ourselves and it is so effective that we encourage our patients to use it as well.

On one side of a sheet of paper, list your meal plan for the week, and on the other side, create the corresponding shopping list. Once your shopping is complete, save this page. After just a few weeks you'll have several plans and corresponding shopping lists all ready to go. When you hit a week that allows no time to create a new plan—and you will surely have those weeks—you can just reach for a plan you've already created.

This simple paper system works great for us and for many others, but you can certainly expand or tweak it. Perhaps you would prefer to use your computer to keep track of your plans and shopping lists. You can even create a folder for each week on your computer that can hold the meal plan, shopping list, and all the recipes for the week.

With a bit of time invested up front in planning and compiling your shopping lists, you will make preparing your meals so much easier down the road. This kind of convenience cannot be underestimated. It's a big part of ensuring that the changes you're making now are sustainable over the long run.

Keep a few things in mind as you make the plan itself:

- Try to plan two or more meals that have ingredients in common. This not only saves time at the grocery store, but it will also help ensure that bunches of leftover herbs, produce, and opened containers of vegetable broth, for instance, don't languish in your refrigerator after you make just one meal with them.

- Make sure that you plan meals you can actually fit into your schedule for the week ahead. A complicated, multipart dish isn't good for a busy weeknight.

- Early in the week or during the weekend, try to cook at least twice what you'll need for that night's dinner so that you have another meal already mostly prepared for later in the week.

- During the weekend, prepare a big batch of grains and/or beans, too, for the week. Both can be easily reheated to serve as part of meals all week, and both make good bases for salads or can be stirred into soups to make them more filling. We'll talk more about this next week.

This extra planning and preparation early in the week means that you'll have a good supply of already-cooked foods ready and waiting to be mixed up in different ways on subsequent nights. We like to also freeze individual meals—kind of like homemade TV dinners. For example, you can put a generous serving of cooked grains or beans in a freezable container and then cover it with stew and freeze. Or bake a full casserole and then divide it into portions and freeze them individually. You can prepare and fully cook a bunch of whole-grain burgers. Put one or more in an individual container and put a portion of the grain-and-stew combination alongside. These containers can be stacked in the freezer easily and removed one at a time for a quick and delicious meal-for-one whenever you need it. The smaller portions defrost more quickly than big batches and these "TV dinners" are as convenient for folks who live alone as they are for people in busy families who sometimes find themselves needing to quickly feed one or a crowd.

The "Food and Mood" Journal

We hear a lot from various sources about how important it is to keep a food diary to track every taste, bite, nibble, dip, and sip we take. There can be some benefits to this, especially if you are trying to lose weight or identify a possible sensitivity to food. But in general we believe that most of us don't want or need to keep such careful records. The most fundamental aspect of Forks Over Knives is that when you eat whole, plant-based foods and you are observing the principles of calorie density (see page 30), then you'll be just fine without tracking anything.

That said, there are some upsides to what we'll call a "food and mood" journal, especially at the beginning of your transition. Once you get the hang of the lifestyle, you won't need it anymore—although if you enjoy keeping it, by all means, do continue. In your journal you can track what you're eating, but also note how you feel physically and emotionally. We're interested in how you feel right around the time you eat and also, especially, how you feel over time. How do you feel when you wake up in the morning? When you are going to bed at night? Note when you feel energetic or satisfied, or, on the other hand, sluggish or bloated. If you experience certain symptoms regularly, such as heartburn, it can be very helpful to note when they occur. If you are suffering from headaches, for instance, do you notice them at any particular time of the day, or after any specific meals? (See the sidebar opposite for some common problems our patients have shared with us over the years.)

Keeping a journal like this is an outstanding way to identify food sensitivities, and it's especially important if you're working with a doctor or other health coach. It's the best first step to discover if any of what you're eating is contributing to discomfort and to help you figure out how to fix it. You may have experienced unpleasant symptoms regularly and perhaps you've assumed that they occur randomly or are discomforts you just have to live with, but a few weeks (or even days) of notes may reveal a pattern that you've missed in the hustle and bustle of life.

If you're trying to lose weight, it can be very useful to track what you consume and when. This not only holds you accountable, but also allows you to measure your progress as well. Do you feel hungry and deprived? Are you not losing the weight you expected to? Did you eat out more often than usual this week? Did you allow yourself more rich options? Is there anything that can be tweaked for your meal plan for next week?

Your journal can be as brief or as detailed as you'd like, but if you're having trouble of any kind, your better bet is to be more detailed until you figure out what's going wrong. Patients sometimes come to us feeling so frustrated because they're sure they're doing everything right and yet they don't feel good or they're not getting the results they hoped for. If something is not going

THE FORKS OVER KNIVES PLAN

Common **Problems** and **Solutions**

Here are a few common ailments people complain of during the first few weeks of their transition to a whole-food, plant-based diet, as well as some ideas for solving them.

PROBLEM: I eat a big breakfast, but I'm always starving by lunch and I find myself eating something that's *not* on the Forks Over Knives plan, which leaves me uncomfortable all afternoon.

SOLUTION: Make sure your breakfast is hearty enough to keep you satisfied until lunch by including a good serving of whole starchy foods, such as potatoes or oats or an abundant quantity of fruit. Also a snack at mid-morning or mid-afternoon can help you head off a derailment. This could be anything—some fruit, a sweet potato and hummus, or a bowl of last night's soup. If you are drinking a fruit-and-veggie smoothie for breakfast and are struggling with satiation, you should consider eating whole foods instead. Eating foods whole rather than blending them often increases satiation.

PROBLEM: I don't feel satisfied with my meals. I am hungry and craving things that I know aren't healthy for me.

SOLUTION: This is where meal planning becomes very important. Write down your meals for the week, including between-meal snacks. Take a good look at the list to make sure you're adding enough flavor, calorie density, and variety to your foods. Try spicing your meals up by adding healthier versions of your favorites, such as our burritos, mashed potatoes, and burgers. A great way to turn off the craving for high-sugar, high-fat, high-sodium foods is to eat some fruit, the natural sweetness of which seems to shut off the drive to eat sugary junk food.

PROBLEM: My energy is low.

SOLUTION: Make sure you are eating enough calories and that you're not eating only raw, leafy vegetables. One of the biggest pitfalls we see is people trying to eat the same portions as they ate on the Standard American Diet. Whole-food, plant-based diets are lower in calorie density so you need to eat until you are comfortably satisfied—which often means bigger portions or more frequent meals.

PROBLEM: It's hard to resist all of the temptations at work. There are *always* doughnuts, chocolates, and candies around!

SOLUTION: Bring your own snacks and desserts to work and make sure that you actually like them and that they are readily available to you. Also make sure you don't allow yourself to get too hungry while those temptations are within reach. It is much harder to make healthy decisions when you are hungry. And, whenever possible, throw out the junk food or avoid the rooms that have them; it is much easier to avoid than to continually resist.

PROBLEM: I am a "foodie." I *love* to cook and eat.

SOLUTION: Great . . . become a *health foodie*! Whole-food, plant-based diets are rich in flavor. And if you love to cook, you'll find fresh inspiration in learning new techniques, being introduced to new ingredients, and discovering new ways to use familiar ingredients and new ones to make familiar foods. There are lots of books and websites out there where you can find recipes for thousands of delicious dishes (see Resources, pages 299–301). Challenge yourself to create any flavor or texture profile you would normally eat using the healthier ingredients you have learned about here.

PROBLEM: I have been on the program for three weeks and I am not losing weight.

SOLUTION: This is a great time to start keeping a food and mood journal (see page 81), if you haven't already, or to step up your use of it if you have. For at least a week or two, include *everything* that goes into your mouth. Make sure to read all the labels on your food to ensure that they have no dairy or oil. Look at what you're eating on the calorie density chart (page 34); you may need to substitute more foods that are lower in calorie density than what you are currently eating (see Calorie Density to Find a Preferred Weight, page 33).

PROBLEM: I am struggling to stick with the program.

SOLUTION: First try to hone in on what exactly is the source of struggle, specifically which need or needs are not being met. For example, if you are overwhelmed because you are thinking of all the things you cannot eat, try addressing this need for pleasure by reversing your thought process and exploring all of the new and delicious recipes at the end of the book. If you are struggling to get out the door easily in the morning and still cook a healthy breakfast, address this need for ease by bringing your dry oatmeal to work with you and simply adding hot water and some fruit when you get there. Finally, be sure to focus on being more intentional with smaller, clearer, affirmative goals. For instance, don't worry about trying to become a chef overnight. Instead, focus on one recipe at a time. And be clear about exactly what you will do and when. Specify that you will always eat a healthy breakfast and will always do your healthy food shopping on Sunday mornings. The keys are being specific and intentional if you want to form healthy new habits long-term, and always trying to identify the strategies and behaviors that will help you meet *all* of your needs.

well, it's almost always because some part of the dietary transition has not yet been fully mastered. The food and mood journal is the first place we look to figure out what's going on. Perhaps the patient has a food sensitivity, or is consuming more fat or sodium than he or she realizes. Whatever it is, the answer will almost surely be in those pages.

Be sure to choose a system for your journal that fits your lifestyle. It can be as low-tech as an ordinary notebook, a specific log designed for the purpose (they are abundant), or you can keep your journal on your computer or mobile device—here, too, you can just keep a running record or you can download programs or applications specifically for the purpose.

EYE ON NUTRITION: CALCIUM AND DAIRY

We're guessing you believe that it's important to get enough calcium and, furthermore, that certain foods, especially milk and other dairy products, are excellent "sources" of it. It's easy to interpret this message—that constant vigilance is necessary to make sure we're getting our calcium—as an implicit warning that we might not otherwise get enough. Heck, they even fortify orange juice with calcium. If they need to do that, it *must* be hard for us to get it naturally, right?

Wrong. Just as with protein (which we discussed last week—see page 68), it is not difficult to get enough calcium—you just need to eat whole, plant-based foods!

Calcium, like iron, magnesium, and copper, is a mineral. It is found in the soil, where it is absorbed into the roots of plants. Animals get their calcium by consuming the mineral-abundant plants and metabolizing that calcium into their bodies. Surprised? That's because we've been so conditioned to think that calcium comes primarily from milk and dairy products that few of us realize it actually comes from the earth and is abundant in *all* whole foods.

Calcium and Strong Bones: The Full Story

Most people think we are doing a good thing for ourselves when we seek out calcium; they believe it will help grow bones when we are young and keep those bones healthy and strong as we age. This is true, to a point. But the full truth is far more nuanced. First, just as with protein, we don't need as much calcium as is implied by all those "Got Milk?" ads. Moreover, how *much* calcium you get isn't as important as where you get it—and how you lose it.

There are two major contributing factors to the leaching of calcium from bones, which leads to their weakening and may increase the risk for osteoporosis: First, consuming a high-sodium diet, and second, consuming a highly acidic diet. The Forks Over Knives diet is naturally low-sodium, as it relies very little on processed foods, which tend to be very high in salt. And as we discussed in Week One, our bodies are alkaline. It is vital that the acidity level of your diet is not so high that your bones must leach calcium to keep your body's alkaline levels balanced. The levels of acidity in plant foods won't draw the calcium from your bones. Eating a whole-food, plant-based diet gives your body the acid/alkaline balance it needs for optimal bone health.

As for the notion that we must consume lots of calcium for good bone health, the evidence does not bear this out. Once a certain threshold has been met—which you will meet eating a whole-food, plant-based diet—the formula for strong bones relies on two other factors entirely:

- First, that you get sufficient vitamin D **from exposure to the sun**. Vitamin D is a key factor in calcium absorption, and the sun is the best way for us to meet our requirement. The key is getting sufficient sun exposure on our bare skin without getting burned (see page 37). The vitamin D in milk is added to it; we do not recommend getting vitamin D from milk or other fortified foods in which the vitamin does not naturally occur.

- Second, that you **practice strength training**. When you lift weights or do resistance exercises you not only build muscle, you stress your bones. This makes them stronger. Walking, jogging, and running are examples of impact exercises that will also help with bone strength.

As with protein, many organizations will suggest that you need to consume a specific amount of calcium per day for strong bones. We do not make any such recommendations because we know that good bone health has nothing to do with hitting an arbitrary number for calcium intake. Furthermore, we fervently believe that when people are instructed to achieve these subjective targets, it creates a skewed notion of what is good nutrition and leads people to make poor food choices.

Calcium is another example of how more of a nutrient is not better. You'll get all the calcium you need from a whole-food, plant-based diet. In fact, as you can see on the chart opposite, adding more calcium to the diet is actually associated with worse bone health.[42] (Calcium supplements have additionally been associated with greater risk of prostate cancer,[43] as well as with death from cardiovascular disease[44] and from all causes.[45]) The important reminder here is that we want to consume our nutrients in the right amounts in the best packages. So rather than focusing on seeking out "enough" calcium, it's much more appropriate to ask how you can best protect your bones and overall health, while also consuming all of the calcium you need. The fiber, carbohydrates, protein, antioxidants, and all the other nutrients that come along with the calcium in plant-based foods are much more essential to your overall good health—including your bones—than any animal-based food.

The Dangers of Bad Packaging

We can believe that you might be having trouble reconciling all of this with everything you've heard about calcium and bones. One of the primary reasons that the National Dairy Council, among others, tells us to drink lots of milk is to protect our bones against degenerative disease like osteoporosis. But the evidence tells a different story. Doubling the protein in the diet increases the loss of calcium into the urine by 50 percent—this can increase both osteopo-

Calcium Consumption Per Capita and Hip Fracture Rates

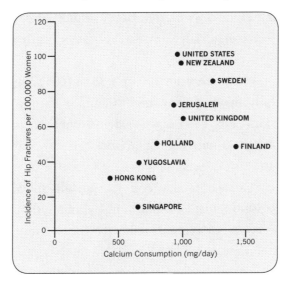

A published report in 1986 by Harvard researcher Mark Hegsted included epidemiological data showing that countries with higher calcium intake had higher rates of hip fractures, a key indicator of osteoporosis. The report concluded that the prevalence of osteoporosis in Western countries is not due to a deficiency of calcium.[46]

rosis and kidney stone risk.[47] Furthermore, an excellent review article on this subject, published in the *American Journal of Clinical Nutrition*, concluded:

Osteoporotic bone fracture rates are highest in countries that consume the most dairy, calcium, and animal protein. Most studies of fracture risk provide little or no evidence that milk or other dairy products benefit bone. Accumulating evidence shows that consuming milk or dairy products may contribute to the risk of prostate and ovarian cancers, autoimmune diseases, and some childhood ailments.[48]

And there are many other concerns about the dairy package. It is high in calories, saturated fat, and cholesterol, and it has no fiber, a trait it shares with other animal-based foods. Consuming calories that don't have fiber will significantly increase your risk of constipation because the bowel requires fiber to function properly. Even worse, dairy proteins seem to specifically impair bowel function.[49]

Dairy increases insulin-like growth factor 1, or IGF-1, a growth hormone that is found naturally in your body and stimulates cell growth.[50] And that means the growth of *all* cells, even unwanted ones such as cancer, specifically breast, prostate, colon, and lung cancers. IGF-1 can also promote premature aging and increase the risk of acne.[51]

Dairy is a common cause of food allergies, especially in children, and there is a possible link between dairy consumption, asthma risk, and lung reactivity. Many people see certain symptoms resolve or lessen very quickly once all dairy is removed from their diet.[52]

We could go on and on, but we think you get the picture. We will add just one more concern, though, because it's one we find particularly worrying. There is a connection between dairy and type 1 diabetes. Studies have shown that the immune system can't differentiate between the amino acids in dairy and insulin-producing cells in our pancreas that look identical. This means that when some people consume dairy products, their immune system attacks both kinds of cells, which can result in so much damage to the pancreatic cells that they no longer produce insulin. The result is type 1 diabetes. In fact, one study showed that the risk of developing type 1 diabetes was more than five times greater in people who consumed three or more glasses of milk per day.[53]

The Takeaway: Calcium and Dairy

We do need calcium, but more isn't necessarily better, and there are many other factors to having strong bones. For example, dairy may be high in calcium, but the package is terrible, with no antioxidants and no fiber, along with high levels of saturated fat, cholesterol, calories, and acidity levels that lead to calcium leaching out of bones and eventually weakening them.

Plant-based foods, on the other hand, have all the calcium we need—and in a package that does a body good!

MAKING IT WORK FOR YOU

Food Addiction and the Myth of Willpower

A week or two into your transition, the degree to which you're already feeling better may make you excited and enthusiastic to continue. This is fantastic! And for some, it's really that simple. They continue transitioning their full diet to whole, plant-based foods, and it just *works* for them. They no longer crave the chocolate cake (or chips, or cheese, or whatever their particular yen was) and their path is relatively smooth from now on.

But many people have a different experience. Not only do they still crave the chocolate cake a few weeks into the transition, they feel terrible about craving it. They tell us that they feel like they *shouldn't* want it, because now they're eating clean and should be "pure." Plus, they worry that they lack will-power, an elusive virtue that we're supposed to be able to access at times like these.

If this sounds familiar, stop beating yourself up for being a perfectly normal person. Cravings and yearning for certain foods are very familiar to most of us. But why is this? Let us start by recognizing what this desire for foods that give us contentment is *not*. It is neither a sign of weakness nor a lack of moral character. Food makes us feel better emotionally and physically by stimulating what we call the "Dopamine Pleasure Cycle." When we eat, the chemical dopamine is released in our brain, which gives us a pleasurable sensation that makes us want to eat more. This is a *survival mechanism* to ensure that we eat.

So you can put all that talk of "willpower" *way* to the back of your mind. Repeat after us: "I am hardwired to crave calorie-rich foods." Generally speaking, the more refined or calorie-dense the food, the greater the dopamine hit.[54] This wiring worked great for our ancestors. When they required energy and they came across various fruits and vegetables, the craving for calorie-rich foods would steer them to choose, say, bananas over leafy vegetables. Bananas, of course, have enough calories per bite to easily make a meal out of them, while the leafy vegetables by themselves do not.

So if we're actually wired this way, when does it become a problem? This natural craving for richer foods was meant for a world where the calorie sources are whole plant foods like bananas—not hamburgers and Twinkies. The latter foods are richer than what was common in our ancestral environment, so the sensory experience feedback we receive is hypernormal; that is, the excitement level is high, but instead of the experience leading us to greater survivability as it was designed to do, it is leading us into a health crisis. The more hamburgers we choose, the more caught in the pleasure cycle we become because more and more dopamine is released. We begin to depend on this artificial heightened level of pleasure—a "high" feeling, if you will—just as if we were taking drugs. The more you're exposed to this feeling, the more you'll turn to these unhealthy foods—crowding out the healthier, more appropriately calorie-dense foods.[55]

Worse yet, we get so caught in the pleasure cycle that we are willing to go to extremes—diet pills, surgery, and ridiculous hours at the gym—to hold on to our ability to indulge in unhealthy eating. This is food addiction. The solution is in your hands: Transition to a whole-food, plant-based diet. The sooner you detach yourself from the Dopamine Pleasure Cycle, the sooner your body will remember how to respond to the real food you were designed to eat.

A great number of Americans are trying to lose weight, yet the number of people who are overweight and obese continues to rise. The problem is that we keep doing the same things over and over again without trying something different. We end up in the familiar "yo-yo" cycle: lose a little weight, keep it off for a while, gain it back, and repeat. This never-ending cycle is exhausting, frustrating, and demoralizing.

As we discussed earlier, mainstream dieting is destined to fail because it emphasizes what we *can't* eat. Restriction and portion control go against our nature to eat to satiation. They rely on "willpower" to ignore real feelings of deprivation and even hunger. But we are not programmed to be hungry! When we restrict, our body receives the message that it is starving. Eventually it fights back, and this is the moment that most of us fall off the "diet" and back into our old eating habits.

Here's how you break the cycle.

Change your lifestyle rather than dieting. Focus on all of the amazing foods you can eat until you are truly satisfied. Eliminate the notion that "will-power" has anything to do with this equation. End restriction and deprivation by choosing whole, plant-based foods. By eating this way you'll be able to eat until satiated without restricting.

Understand your cravings. What you're feeling is real. However, as we'll discuss in more detail next week, you don't have to give in to it the same way that you might have before. Instead, figure out a way to resolve the cravings within the scope of your new lifestyle. Ask yourself, did you take away every-thing that gave you pleasure before your transition? You need balance in your meal plan, so if you're feeling deprived, it's important to address it. Cravings for unhealthy foods tend to pass over time as you transition to finding healthy foods that you love. This is called *neurological adaptation;* you're used to being hyperstimulated, so ordinary stimulation seems bland. There will probably be bumps at first. Our friend Doug Lisle, PhD, describes this as being a little like coming indoors after you've been out in the bright sun for a while. Until you acclimate, it seems terribly dark; you may even smack into the furniture. But with a little time your eyes adjust and everything becomes quite clear. Simi-larly, if you are used to a diet of high-calorie-density foods, the change to low-calorie-density foods will require a period of adjustment. Over time, by eating foods that are natural to us, your body will get used to the lower, more normal levels of dopamine stimulation and this will begin to feel good.

Don't panic that you're craving unhealthy foods; just take a deep breath, look in your well-stocked pantry, and ask yourself, "What *can* I eat?" If you're craving something sweet, for example, try fruit or a fruit-based ice "cream" from this book (page 284); or if you're craving something crunchy, try baked pita chips with hummus made from navy beans (page 168), lentils (page 261), or chickpeas and sun-dried tomatoes (page 263).

Don't go hungry. This is perhaps the most important of these because this is when we make some of our worst food choices and why meal planning is so necessary. If you feel hungry, make sure you're eating at meals until you are comfortably full. If you know you're going to have a particularly busy day, pack snacks to eat between appointments.

Finally, give your body time to adjust to its new reality. Little by little you'll learn how to respond to the clues your body is giving you to tell you what it needs. We don't want you ever to feel deprived. There has never been an easier time to go plant-based than now when such abundant resources are available to help you. A world of nourishing foods that taste amazing and satisfy you is here, waiting for you to discover it. You can begin with the recipes in this book, of course, and then check out the Resources on page 299 for a list of our favorite sources for recipes and information.

GETTING PERSONAL

After so many years of cooking the same meals for my family, there was a definite learning curve to finding new "regular" dinners that we could all eat. Now that there are new dinners in the repertoire, it's a snap. The more I eat this way, the more I want to. I'm still baffled when people ask what I eat . . . like I'm depriving myself? I feel like I have more choices now than ever!

—Melinda Wester, 50, office manager, Lexington, KY

I have a small stable of go-to recipes. I have gotten more intuitive in cooking plant-based dishes, just from experience. Familiarity and practice will continue to make it easier and easier to continue to eat better and cleaner over time. Also, I do notice my tastes changing. I'm pretty sure I like things now that I wouldn't have liked at the start of this journey.

—Jennifer Starbuck, 45, stay-at-home mom, Murrieta, CA

No meat was easy, but no dairy was a real challenge. . . . Wow. I had no idea I was so addicted. I feel so much cleaner and alive.

—Amy Janssens, 37, small business owner, Petoskey, MI

I don't like what I feel like when I do eat the bad foods. I get an upset stomach and even constipation if I eat like I used to. Now when I think of going off the plan, I try to remember how bad the foods make me feel and that usually keeps me on track.

—Sandy Lodyga, 39, teacher, Valrico, FL

I no longer have the cravings I used to experience (like stopping on the way home from work at In-N-Out Burger or eating a bunch of Lay's potato chips). I like to cook and it's become a bit of a hobby exploring new recipes. My children have jumped right in and eat what I make. Both have seen their just-beginning acne slow down.

—Bonnie Safyurtlu, 46, regulatory affairs—pharmaceuticals, Irvine, CA

Cooking is easy. Brown rice, potatoes, and whole-grain pasta are cheap and easy to store and cook. The delicious food that I could eat without restraint, knowing that it was all good for me. Also, I find that I have lost cravings for many foods I used to love.

—Ben Hall, 41, nurse, Haywards Heath, West Sussex, United Kingdom

When you eat poorly, you feel poorly. Eating healthy makes me lighter and happier. Why would I want to go back? It seems like self-punishment, and I don't want to punish my body.

—Erica Kelsey, 35, government relations, Toronto, Canada

WEEK THREE: **The Forks Over Knives Dinner**

CHAPTER 6

As you launch the third week of your transition, you may be reaping some early benefits from your new lifestyle. Perhaps you have a bit more energy, or you're not experiencing "food hangovers" as often as you did previously. Some people tell us that a couple of weeks into their transition they notice changes in areas of their lives they never before considered to be diet-related. They're sleeping better, perhaps, or are thirsty less often, or have greater energy at the times of day they used to drag. Many people love the freedom they gain in a kitchen free of animal-based food—with no more worrying about cross-contamination of cutting boards or refrigerator shelves and drawers. In grocery stores they can bypass the fish, meat, and deli counters entirely and instead spend more time in the colorful produce section.

On the other hand, if you're not yet feeling anything like this, don't despair—and absolutely don't give up. Your transition is your own, and you must be sensitive to your personal needs. This week in addition to changing your dinner, we'll talk in more detail about how to cook delicious, healthy food the Forks Over Knives way. We'll also unravel the mysteries of fat and oil. And we'll pick up where we left off in last week's Making It Work For You discussion about food addiction and willpower with a deeper examination of deprivation and cravings. These significant themes can be persistent in the early days

THE FORKS OVER KNIVES PLAN

of the transition. It's important to understand the physiology and psychology that cause them in order to rise above them and make the whole-food, plant-based lifestyle *your* lifestyle.

But first things first: This week when you make your meal plan, redesign your nightly dinners just as you have your two other daily meals. Consider what you usually eat. If your dinner plate typically holds the standard "protein, car-bohydrate, vegetable" trinity, it's time to expand and merge your perceptions of each of those components until you're able to see a plate of *food* instead of food groups and nutrients. We offer many great recipes in the back of the book for meals that blur the line between lunch, dinner, and even breakfast. This is how we eat, and we encourage you to eat the same way. However, it is also true that many of the people we talk to and treat regard the evening meal as the most elaborate of the day for a variety of reasons. If you identify with this point of view, then we've got you covered: Polenta Casserole with Cilan-tro Chutney (page 228), Curried Twice-Baked Potatoes (page 222), Spaghetti with White Bean Alfredo (page 235), Tex-Mex Bean and Cornbread Casserole (page 219), and Potato-Vegetable Chowder (page 204) are all substantial and satisfying dishes. (Also see the Resources on page 299 for great books and online sources for recipes.) And don't forget that this is the time to clean out your old dinner standbys if you didn't do it during Week One's pantry purge (see page 58).

If you've read every page of this book up to now, including the discussions on nutrients in the introduction and protein and calcium in Weeks One and Two, you understand that the complete package of whole, plant-based foods on your Forks Over Knives plate will provide the nutrition your body needs to flourish. So just remember that as long as you are eating fruits, vegetables, tubers, whole grains, and legumes in sufficient quantity, you'll be more than fine. In fact, you will thrive!

LET'S GET PRACTICAL:
COOKING THE FORKS OVER KNIVES WAY

Whether cooking is your passion or you consider it a last resort to be undertaken only when your favorite restaurants are inexplicably closed, a few basic strategies will simplify the most fundamental aspects of cooking the Forks Over Knives way.

Cooking in Bulk

One of the best things about cooking for your new lifestyle is how much of your daily meals and snacks can be prepared in advance. As we mentioned last week, try to spend a little time once a week making one big pot of beans and another big pot of rice or another grain. In addition, we often bake a bunch of white or sweet potatoes. All of these will keep in the refrigerator for up to a week and none of them require much active time in the kitchen. These items will be the backbone of your meals all week long. A few times each week, we steam a pound or two of our favorite vegetables—green beans, broccoli, cauliflower, carrots, or whatever looks good at the store or market. They'll keep in the refrigerator for several days.

This is what we do most weekends to get ahead, and it makes an enormous difference all week long. With a few sauces, dressings, and condiments on hand, we can pull together a delicious, nourishing meal in minutes using any combination of these refrigerator staples. You can chop up baked potatoes and some vegetables and toss with a sauce for a big one-dish meal, or sauté an onion and some garlic, add one or two already-cooked vegetables, cook just a minute or two to reheat, and serve over rice or another grain. Plus, any of these items can be wrapped in a corn tortilla, stirred into soup or stew, or mixed with pasta and sauce to make it more filling and satisfying.

Cooking Without Oil or Some Other Old Standbys

By now you've probably heard howls of "No oil? Are you joking!?" from your friends and family—or you may well have had these thoughts yourself. We've certainly heard this a lot over the years, and truth be told, we don't know what all the fuss is about. It is not at all difficult to cook delicious food without oil. In fact, most people find they enjoy their food more without the grease. Plus, between the missing oil and the missing animal products, you're not only eating healthier, you're cooking cleaner. This means that the after-meal washing up is a whole lot easier, which we think you'll agree is a very good thing.

We'll talk more about *why* we exclude oil in our Eye on Nutrition section below. For now we'll focus on *how* to cook without oil. The first thing to consider is your choice of pans. We use primarily nonstick pots and pans in our kitchen, but these are not mandatory. If you prefer to avoid Teflon-coated nonstick pans, you can certainly use good-quality, heavy-bottomed stainless-steel pans. Enamel-coated cast iron and ceramic titanium are other good options. Above all, it is best to invest in pans that are good quality, not thin or shoddily made. It is far better to have three or four excellent pans—a small saucepan, a large saucepan, and a skillet and/or a sauté pan would be our choices, along with well-fitting lids—than it is to have ten inferior ones. And fewer good pans are likely to cost the same as, if not less than, a larger number of second-rate ones.

Once you have the proper pans, the only thing you really need to know about stovetop cooking is how to sauté and stir-fry without oil or butter. This is easy: We use vegetable broth or water instead. The trick is to not use too much liquid, which can lead to steamed, not browned, vegetables. The recipes in this book demonstrate the different ways we use this technique. If you're cooking without a recipe, or are trying to adapt a recipe to be oil-free, we advise you to place whatever you're sautéing in the pan over the heat and let it cook for a few minutes until it begins to sizzle and brown a bit around the edges. When the vegetables or grains begin to stick, add the liquid just 1 or 2 tablespoons at a time and use a wooden spatula or other pan-safe tool to loosen the ingredients from the bottom and redistribute them evenly around the pan. Cook until the liquid has evaporated. Continue this process, adding small bits of liquid when the ingredients begin to stick to the pan and letting the liquid cook off each time until your ingredients have reached whatever stage you're looking for (translucent, softened, crisp-tender, browned, etc.).

When we bake, we use pureed fruit such as unsweetened applesauce, dates, or crushed pineapple in place of oil or butter, as we do in the Chewy Lemon-Oatmeal Cookies (page 278). The fruit contributes moisture and flavor to baked goods that traditionally rely on added fat for these qualities along with a nice touch of natural sweetness. We will occasionally use a small amount of sugar when baking—as in the Apple Crisp (page 287)—keeping in mind the calorie contribution of this added sugar will be minimal.

The thing to remember is that the more you cook the Forks Over Knives way, the more comfortable you will become with these new techniques and ingredients. The creaminess and richness you once associated with milk, eggs, or butter will now come from other, healthier sources. We make delicious, creamy mashed potatoes (page 180), for example, by mixing in a small amount of pureed cashews. We use small amounts of plant-based milk in some recipes. Unsweetened rice, almond, hazelnut, or soy milks are all good options, so go with the one you prefer. (Whichever you use, make sure it is unsweetened and does not contain a flavor you are not looking for in the recipe. For example, a vanilla-flavored or sweetened plant-based milk doesn't taste so good in chowder.)

Another of our favorite standbys is nutritional yeast, which provides that wonderful, savory "umami" taste that many of us crave in dishes like the Big Breakfast Burrito (page 151) and Sweet Potato Mac and Cheese (page 236). To add smoky richness to dishes like Potato Enchiladas (page 220), not to mention any beans, greens, or stews, make sure you have a smoked spice in your cabinet—smoked paprika and ground chipotle are two great choices. Additionally, many stores now carry their own mixed spice blends (which often include a smoked variety). A dash or two of any of these can be tasty while still allowing the natural flavors of the primary, plant-based ingredients to come through; we especially like to stir them into our favorite recipes for hummus and salsa to quickly and easily change their flavor profile.

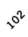
That's it! As you can see, there's no great mystery to cooking this way. Yes, the results will be different from what you are used to—but different is what you want. This sort of different is definitely *better* in that you'll now enjoy bright, fresh flavors and also vastly improved health.

If cooking the Forks Over Knives way seems daunting or even radical right now, trust that the more you eat this way, the more you will actually crave these new foods. You are retraining and reprogramming not only your palate but also your physiological response to food (see Making It Work For You, below, for more on this). What might seem like tremendous change right now will soon be second nature to you. Take a good look at the well-stocked kitchen (pages 59–65) for a full list of fresh, dried, and frozen ingredients that you'll soon come to think of not merely as *substitutions* for what you're no longer eating but the tried-and-true *staples* of your delicious whole-food, plant-based diet. This is not a diet of deprivation; you don't have to avoid satisfying flavors to be healthy.

Now that we've talked a bit about various ingredients and alternatives for you to consider as you transition to a whole-food, plant-based diet, we want to remind you of the delicious things you *will* eat—many of which may be new to you. As we discussed last week and will touch on again this week in Making It Work For You, it's very important to understand where feelings of deprivation come from. It's equally important to learn how to tend to these feelings when they present themselves.

This isn't merely about finding healthier alternatives to your favorite desserts (which you can do on pages 275–287). Potatoes and legumes, as well as foods like dips, spreads, sauces, and dressings (pages 258–274), can help create more satisfying meals. Furthermore, go ahead and seek out the Forks Over Knives versions of your favorite casseroles, pizzas, lasagnas, and even mashed potatoes and gravy. There are delicious recipes for every one of these dishes in this book.

Cooking With Friends

It is entirely possible to make this transition on your own—although we hasten to add that you never have to be completely alone if you take advantage of the fabulous online communities available to everyone, all the time. The Forks Over Knives website and Facebook page are great places to begin to discover the world of like-minded and inspiring people out there ready to share recipes, offer tips for getting through rough patches, and generally just cheer one another on.

That said, it's always nicest to have some in-person companionship along the way. One of the best methods to nurture this is to create a buddy system for cooking and sharing meals. Bring together one or more friends and neighbors who are transitioning or already living the whole-food, plant-based way. Divvy up some or all of the week's dinners, assigning each member of your group a night on which he or she prepares enough for everyone. You can choose to eat together some nights, or you can simply arrange to drop off or pick up the food before the meal.

This is a phenomenal way to get motivated—it's more exciting and fun to cook when there is camaraderie. Plus, each week you can share with one another the recipes and lessons gleaned in your own kitchens. Communal learning is often its own incentive, when a group of mutually motivated folks root for and support one another. It becomes more than just sharing the cooking a few nights a week, although that in and of itself can be a pretty wonderful advantage. It's a way to ensure a successful transition and sustained lifestyle for all of you. Next week we'll talk a bit about adapting the buddy system to the workplace.

EYE ON NUTRITION: FATS

Some fats are necessary in our diet. Consuming oil and processed foods as a means to get these, however, is unnecessary, and even harmful. Every whole plant food has fat, and there's no evidence that we need any more fat

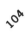
than what occurs naturally in a low-fat, whole-food, plant-based diet. Just as is the case with protein and calcium, we should not target specific foods to get enough of a particular kind of fat.

There are two types of fat: unsaturated and saturated. Most foods contain both of these types of fat; whichever is present in the larger quantity determines how we refer to that fat, and by extension, that food. The unsaturated fats come in two forms, either monounsaturated or polyunsaturated. The two fats that we must get from food sources are the two polyunsaturated fats, omega-3 and omega-6, which only plants can make. We call these "essential fatty acids" because our bodies can't make them and so it is *essential* that we eat them.

Omega-3 and omega-6 fatty acids appear to be involved in a variety of important bodily functions, including cell membrane stabilization, nervous system function, immune system function, and blood clotting, as well as impacting triglyceride levels, blood pressure, inflammation, cancer, and heart disease. Although they are both essential, you have probably heard a lot more often that you need to seek out omega-3. This is *not* because it is more essential than omega-6. Instead, it is because, in general, these two essential fatty acids should be consumed in a healthy ratio to each other. Studies are not clear *exactly* what that ratio should be, but we do know that the Standard American Diet is significantly skewed in such a way that we get an excess of omega-6. This excess consumption of omega-6 impairs the absorption of omega-3.[56] The answer, however, is not simply that you need to eat more omega-3 fats. The answer is to eliminate or minimize processed and animal-based foods and instead eat a whole-food, plant-based diet, which we know in most cases restores a healthy omega-6 to omega-3 balance and, more important, leads to positive health outcomes. And isn't *that* what we care about most?

You may yet wonder how much *total* essential fatty acids you should eat. If 1 to 3 percent of your calories come from the essential fats, you'll be in great shape. Adequate omega-3 intake specifically is 1.1 g for adult women and 1.6 g for adult men.[57] That's ¼ to ⅓ teaspoon per day. If you meet all your caloric needs with a low-fat, whole-foods diet full of fruits, vegetables, whole grains, and legumes, you will easily consume enough essential fatty acids *and* those fatty acids will be in good balance to each other. Note that while walnuts and flax- and chia seeds are whole plant foods with higher concentrations of essential fatty acids, there's no evidence that you actually need to eat these foods to get the proper amount of any kind of fat. Most whole plant foods have small amounts of essential fats. Over the course of a day full of these foods you will achieve the needed amounts—which aren't that much to begin with. In fact, it is significantly more important to worry about not consuming excess fat than it is to worry about consuming sufficient omega-3.

The Problem with Eating Fish for Omega-3 Fatty Acids

As for the oft-repeated pronouncement that fish is a great source of omega-3, it is true that fish contain concentrated amounts of these essential fatty acids (which they have only because they get them from the *plants* that they eat). However, there are several significant problems with consuming fish for omega-3:

- A convincing case has never been made that we need such concentrated amounts of omega-3.

- An omega-3-rich "health" food like salmon is 40 percent fat. This is too much. And two-thirds of the fat is nonessential, a type of fat that is of no use and is harmful in this high amount.

- Remember, too, that food is never a single nutrient; food is comprised of "packages" of nutrients and substances. And the fish package is not a good one. For example, fish contains the same heart-unhealthy cholesterol that red meat contains; is high in acids that lead to bone loss and increase the risk of osteoporosis; lacks fiber; and is often tainted with contaminants such as mercury and polychlorinated biphenyls (PCBs).

Fish: An Animal that Swims

We are always surprised by how many people continue to think that fish is beneficial and important to include in the diet, even long after they become convinced that mammals are not health foods. Much of this perception stems from periodic reports that some study or another has found that fish is "heart healthy" or "good for our brains." In our review of these studies, time and again we find data is misinterpreted and faulty conclusions are drawn from otherwise reasonable research. Unfortunately, such misinterpretations have occurred so frequently that a false narrative has developed.

One of the most egregious examples of this phenomenon is the poor interpretation of the famous Okinawan Centenarian Study, published in 2007. In this twenty-five-year study, sponsored by the Japanese Ministry of Health, researchers examined the diet and lifestyle of hundreds of elderly Japanese renowned for their longevity and relative freedom from the chronic ailments that typically plague Westerners in their later years. The fundamental message of the study is sound: Diet and lifestyle matter. We take issue, though, with the common conclusion that many draw from this research; that is, that the *fish* in the Okinawans' diet was a major contributing factor to their long life spans and extraordinary good health. Now here's a fact that may surprise you: Only 1 percent of the calories consumed by the Okinawans came from fish; the vast majority of their diet—69 percent—came from sweet potatoes![58] So the indelible perception that the Okinawans consumed a fish-heavy diet is demonstrably false.

The practice of misinterpreting data is not unusual. Studies from Mediterranean countries follow this pattern, too. The benefits of a diet high in fruits, vegetables, and whole grains frequently get credited to small amounts of fish in the diet (just like they are often credited to olive oil and wine). What is happening here? We have meaningful long-term studies presented by the researchers with care, which are then pored over by individuals or organizations who cherry-pick data, often to reinforce a specific agenda. The big picture is ignored in favor of subjective claims and reporting, and the public receives false takeaway messages like "Eat more fish!"

The bottom line with fish is that it's an animal that swims in water. As our friend and teacher Dr. John McDougall likes to say, "A muscle is a muscle, whether it comes from a chicken, cow, or fish." In other words, the nutrient profile of all animal products—i.e., high in fat, acid, and cholesterol, and low in fiber and carbohydrates—is as true for fish as it is for beef and other meats. In fact, although fish is often marketed as a wise, "heart-healthy" food choice, it has as much cholesterol as beef, chicken, and pork. When it comes to nutrition, you've heard us say to focus not on single nutrients but the whole package of nutrition. Similarly, when we look at studies of populations and what they eat, we should not look at individual variables, but rather examine the entire big picture. In doing so, we see the message is consistent: "Eat more plants!"

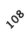

THE FORKS OVER KNIVES PLAN

With fish, as we've seen before with other animal-based foods, making food choices based on individual nutrients gets us into trouble.

The Myth of "Healthy" Oils

We are baffled that certain oils are presented as "health" foods. Olive oil is *not* a health food. Neither is coconut, grape seed, flaxseed, or any other oil you've heard you must endeavor to add to your diet because it's good for you. Sure, if you replace some or all of the butter in your diet with vegetable oil, you may do a little bit better, but that's not at all the same as doing *well*. Oil is a bad idea because it is highly refined and its nutritional package is inadequate.

How is it that we know that processed sugars are junk foods, yet we've allowed ourselves to be convinced that certain oils are somehow good for us? Oil follows essentially the same model as processed sugar, which is also pressed from plants. Think about what oil is: fat—and nothing but fat. All the nutrients, including protein, carbohydrates, vitamins, minerals, fiber, and water, have been thrown away. Oil of any kind has more calories per gram than any other food we know. And without any fiber or water in it, oil lacks the bulk to convey to your senses how many calories you have eaten; this virtually guarantees you will consume more calories at the meal than you need. So we ask you: Why would you waste calories on something that has no nutrients in it other than fat? And why would anyone believe that highly concentrated fat is healthy?

So let's look at where the "good oil" hype came from. Its origins lay in data collected in the 1960s that showed the people on the island of Crete at that time had the lowest all-cause mortality rates over twenty years when compared to people in other Mediterranean countries. A main contributing factor was their diet, which included some animal products and a little bit of olive oil, but otherwise consisted primarily of fruits, vegetables, and whole grains.[59] In the years since then, unfortunately, the phrase "Mediterranean diet" has become synonymous primarily with olive oil. What subsequent researchers—and marketers—took from those early studies was that olive oil was the Holy Grail. But it never was.

More recently, the largest Mediterranean diet study to date looked at 22,000 adults aged 20 to 86. Researchers found that olive oil produced no significant reduction in overall death rates. The real benefits of the Mediterranean diet were its high intake of vegetables, fruit, legumes, and whole grains. They noted that there was moderate fish intake and the intake of meat and dairy was low.[60] Dr. Alice Lichtenstein of the Human Nutrition Research Center on Aging at Tufts University, one of the nation's top nutrition scientists, observed, "If the main message that Americans get is to just increase their olive or canola oil consumption that's unfortunate, because they will increase their caloric intake and they are already getting too many calories. *What they need to do is eat more fruits, vegetables, and legumes,* and fewer foods rich in saturated fats" [emphasis added].

And as for the very real dangers? *All oils* have a negative impact on blood vessels and promote heart disease.[61] Furthermore, they may also lead to increased bleeding through thinning of the blood; negative effects on lung function and oxygen exchange; suppression of certain immune system functions; and increased risk of cancer.[62] Not to mention that excess calories from fat get stored *as* fat, no matter what type of fat calories you consume.

The Takeaway: Fats

All you have to do is eat the right foods without targeting any specific one as a good source for this or that kind of fat. You'll get *all* the essential fats you need, and in just the right proportions to support good health. Once again, nature has it figured out perfectly!

MAKING IT WORK FOR YOU

Dealing with Deprivation and Cravings

In Weeks One and Two we discussed how so many of us feel like the only way to be successful—at losing weight, getting our cholesterol under control, lowering our blood pressure, and so on—is to be deprived. If you've ever tried to achieve success in any of these or similar areas while eating the Standard American Diet, you almost certainly engaged in restriction of some kind. And if you've restricted, it's likely that at least once you found yourself pulled between two opposing sides of an endless loop. On one side are the feelings of guilt for eating foods you shouldn't when dieting. On the other are feelings of deprivation caused by staying away from beloved foods. These aren't feelings of the purely emotional kind (although that certainly plays a part in cravings, as we discuss below). These feelings have a physiological basis, and they are brought on when portion control—eating less—interferes with our leptin cycle.

Leptin is the hormone released by your fat cells when they sense that you have taken in enough food. When this happens, your hunger signals shut down. You no longer feel hungry; you stop eating. Nice and simple, right? Sure, except when your hunger signals have been radically distorted by restrictive portion control. Your body *knows* you haven't consumed enough calories so it tells you to eat more by making you feel hungry. Eating less leads to your body releasing less satiation-signaling leptin. Now your appetite increases, right along with your cravings.[63] You can resist for a while, perhaps, but you're fighting your body's natural instinct to get the correct number of calories and avoid starvation. This is not a fight you are likely to win over the long run because your body thinks you'll die if you don't get enough calories.

Eventually, you'll need to feed your body more, and when your body thinks it's starving you will be drawn to the most calorie-dense, usually fattening, foods. Many people also binge at this point, all of which can lead to a demoralizing weight gain and a failure to achieve good health.

The leptin cycle is only one part of the problem. Another is the Dopamine

Pleasure Cycle that we talked about last week (see page 91). The more highly stimulating high-fat, high-calorie foods you eat, the more your body craves them and the less satisfying healthy foods are by comparison. Embarking on a restricting diet after years of eating this way can cause a highly unpleasant physical crash similar to what happens when one suddenly eliminates caffeine. You feel tired, anxious, miserable, and desperate for another hit.

In short, "Eat less!" and its frequent companion, "Exercise more!" are not consistent with a sustainable lifestyle. The only sure way to conquer this vicious cycle is to avoid it in the first place. And here's the good news: Forks Over Knives is not about restriction. It is about resetting your physiology so that your body relearns what is normal. As we discussed on page 93, this neurological adaptation is like acclimating to an inside room after being in sunlight.

Feeling some cravings for unhealthy foods as your body acclimates during the first couple of weeks of the transition is to be expected. Last week we asked you to repeat these words: "I am hardwired to crave calorie-rich foods." Your hardwiring hasn't changed—nor will it. The period you're in now is reminding and retraining your body to respond normally to normal stimuli. It'll take a little time, but keep at it and your body *will* learn. You're reintroducing it to its natural state.

If, after several weeks, you're still experiencing regular and acute cravings, it's time to stop and assess. Take a really good look at what you're eating and check in on whether you are meeting your basic needs for ease, health, and pleasure. Are you trying to survive on "big" green salads? You need to make your plate of food more calorie dense—add beans, grains, or potatoes to that green salad. Perhaps you find cooking this way too time-consuming. Are you trying to prepare overly complicated meals? Please simplify—you are craving the *convenience* of to-go food more than the food itself. Check out the recipes in this book; many can be made very quickly and easily. And make sure your refrigerator is *always* stocked with steamed or baked vegetables and at least one big container of beans or grains—preferably both. Equally important are some condiment foods that make you feel satisfied; dips and dressings, or

THE FORKS OVER KNIVES PLAN

small amounts of nuts, seeds, or avocado are all items that can quickly and easily transform a plate of, say, beans and steamed vegetables into a delicious and satisfying meal.

Picture this scenario: Since your transition to a whole-food, plant-based diet, you've passed the fast-food joint that used to be a regular part of your life twenty times without stopping. But on the twenty-first time, you stop. Why? It's not because something changed in the fast-food joint. It's because something changed in *you*. Maybe you had a lousy day, or you ate nothing but carrot sticks for lunch, or you did a harder-than-usual workout an hour before. Whatever it is, the answer lies within *you*. And it's not about your lack of willpower; it's about your lack of attention to your basic needs. So forgive yourself. Then figure out how you'll change your meal plan or your habits to let you pass that fast-food joint without stopping ever again.

GETTING PERSONAL

I also noticed a new feeling of calm—I had not noticed feeling particularly stressed before changing my diet, but the more relaxed, calm feeling I had in everyday situations was great. I find that rather than feeling deprived, I feel excited to find new recipes. I often use spices or ingredients that I hadn't previously used. . . . I experience zero guilt when eating, and I eat whenever I feel hungry. I have a very positive attitude, knowing that I can maintain this lifestyle and my weight without putting so much effort into tracking every morsel of food, or ever feeling unsatisfied.

—Michelle Williams, 46, stay-at-home mom, Westbrook, ME

In the past few years, social media sites have offered a sort of camaraderie among vegans. I like feeling good, and I don't want to *not* feel good. Remembering that helps me stick to this way of eating.

—Ann Osborn, 49, housewife, Baltimore, MD

I started by trying to make tofu taste like fish or chicken during the first three months. Now that my tastes have changed I find that I hardly use tofu. I can't imagine eating anything that "tastes" like meat. I don't even care for the meat substitutes.

—Brenda Rawlings, 59, Respiratory Therapist, Granite City, IL

I cook extra beans or grains and freeze packets so they are ready for a recipe. I make up packets to freeze of stuffed cabbage, soups, veggie burgers . . . so I'll be prepared for busy days when I can't spend time cooking.

—Andrea Levin Parnes, 62, piano teacher, San Jose, CA

I have way more energy; no more midday naps. I am able to eat all the carbs I can get my hands on. I've lost seven pounds in two weeks without even trying.

—Michael Mason, 40, sales representative, San Diego, CA

When questions are asked, I try to keep my answers brief and refer them to websites or books to read. For me, this is easy to stick with. I love the way I eat. I love the way I feel.

—Marylu Thomas, 59, radiographer, Easton, PA

It is now easier than ever to maintain my healthy weight, and I have never eaten so much in my life. It's amazing.

—Lisa Nelson, 31, self-employed, Moreno Valley, CA

CHAPTER 7

WEEK FOUR:
Fine-Tuning Your Lifestyle

You made it! We are so happy that you are ready to begin your fourth and final transition week. We're not making any big changes to your meal plan this week since you're already planning seven full days of plant-based foods every week. The final week of your transition is about reflection, assessment, and strategizing for long-term success (and, if necessary, removing any last vestiges of your old diet from your pantry and kitchen; see page 58). This week we cover the topics we find most relevant for moving beyond your transition and into the rest of your life. We'll give you some road-tested advice on managing your diet when eating in restaurants, while traveling, or when you are a guest in someone else's home. We explain carbohydrates and their important role in a healthy diet. And finally, we tackle how to handle sticky social situations when you find yourself at the receiving end of too many questions about your lifestyle.

But first, we want to fine-tune your weekly meal plan. Take a look at last week's plan, as well as your food and mood journal (see page 81). Make sure that the food you are consuming is whole and plant based. We understand that over the last three weeks you may not have followed a flawlessly straight line from whatever you were eating before to plant-based diet perfection today. That's okay—life doesn't go in a straight line. Use this extra week to clean

THE FORKS OVER KNIVES PLAN

up around the edges and eliminate whatever vestiges of your old eating habits still remain. One big pitfall is often the food you eat on the run, between meals, or any other time when you're not sitting down to a full meal.

We're not big advocates for scheduled daily snacks because for most people every day is different. Some days you may not be hungry at all between your meals, while on others you may have a voracious appetite—perhaps because of a strenuous workout. Or maybe you regularly find that no matter how much you eat at your meals, you need a little something extra at some point during the day. There can be all sorts of reasons for this: You may have a speedy metabolism or you're an active person or you just haven't figured out how much you need to eat at each meal to keep you satiated until your next one. The point is that no matter what the reason for hunger outside of meal times, the answer is to make sure you're eating the right kinds of foods at meals and, if necessary, in between meals.

We've found that at this point in the transition some people still feel constrained by residual notions of what they previously considered to be a "proper" breakfast, lunch, dinner, or snack. Remember, though, that when you live a whole-food, plant-based lifestyle, lunch can be a large bowl of fruit and breakfast can be a baked potato with steamed vegetables and hummus. Even snacks don't have to be typical snack food. Sometimes we have a second serving of lunch for a snack. Your new lifestyle is about freedom—freedom from worrying about getting "enough" individual nutrients; freedom from the compulsion to make sure your dinner plate conforms to the protein-carb-vegetable template; and freedom from the destructive fallacy that you must restrict and deprive yourself in order to eat healthfully and lose weight.

At the end of this week you will have completed your Forks Over Knives transition—now all you need to do is get out there and enjoy it!

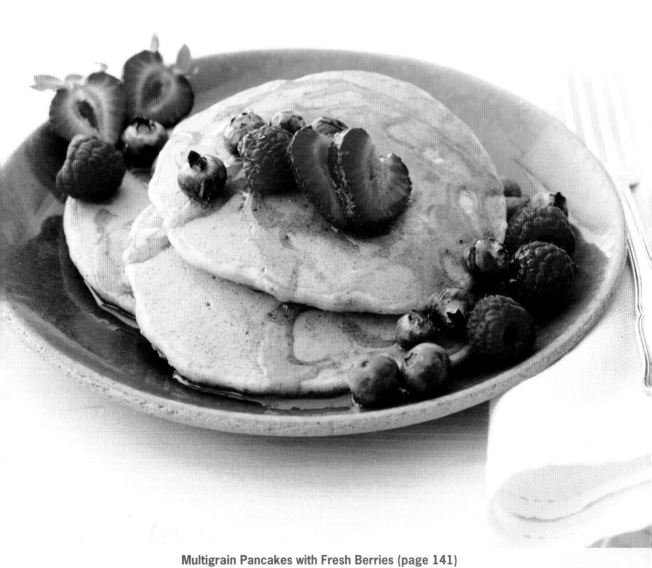

Multigrain Pancakes with Fresh Berries (page 141)

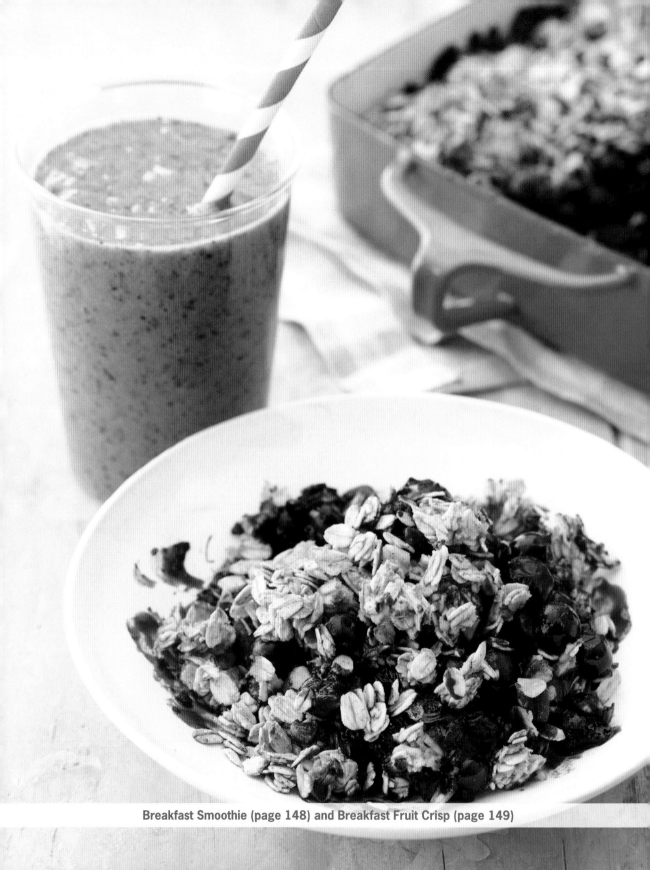

Breakfast Smoothie (page 148) and Breakfast Fruit Crisp (page 149)

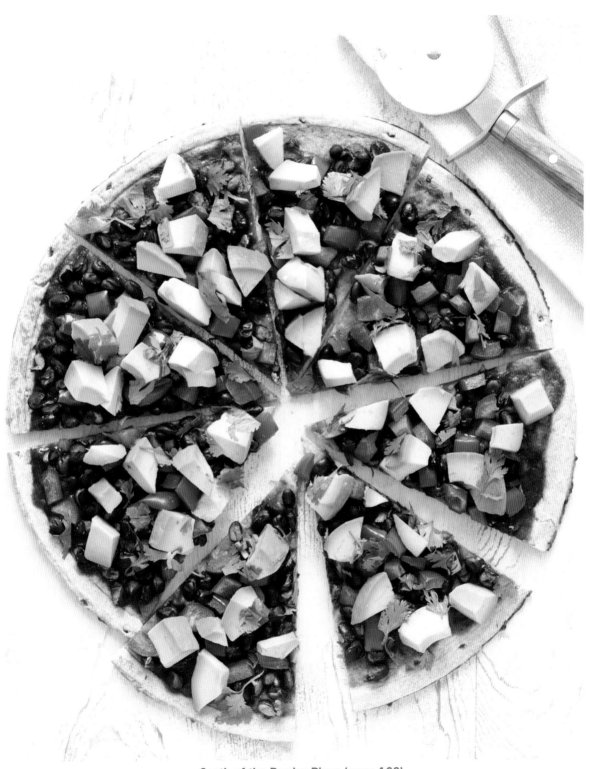

South-of-the-Border Pizza (page 163)

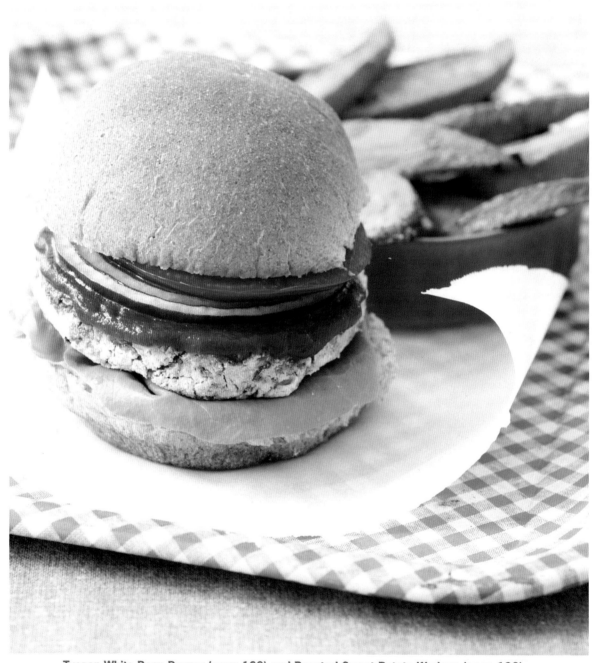

Tuscan White Bean Burger (page 166) and Roasted Sweet Potato Wedges (page 186)

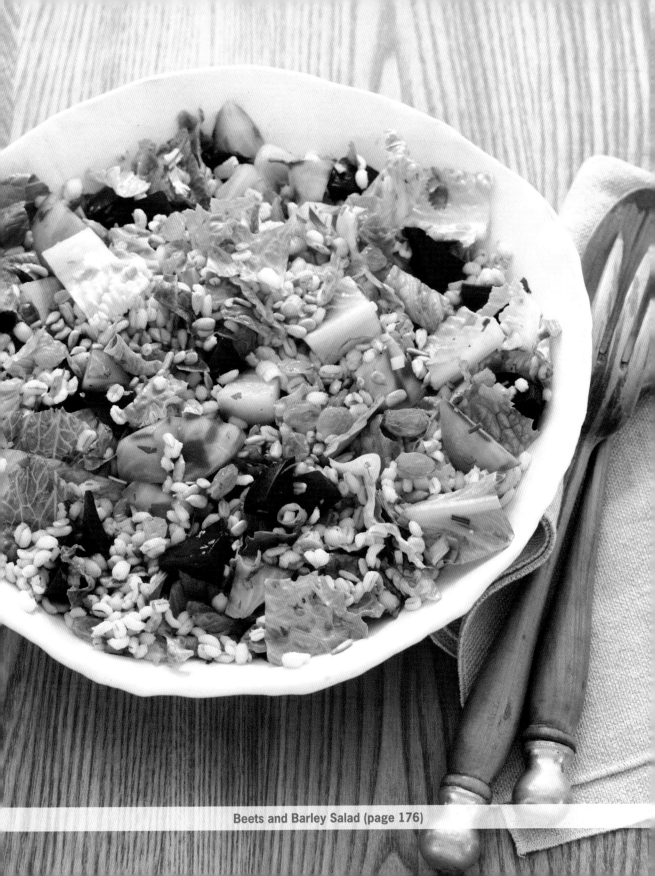

Beets and Barley Salad (page 176)

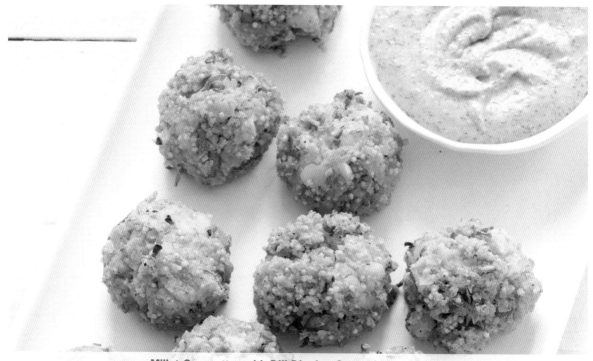

Millet Croquettes with Dill Dipping Sauce (page 182)

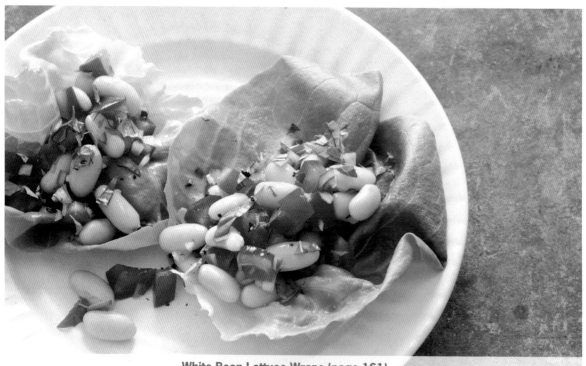

White Bean Lettuce Wraps (page 161)

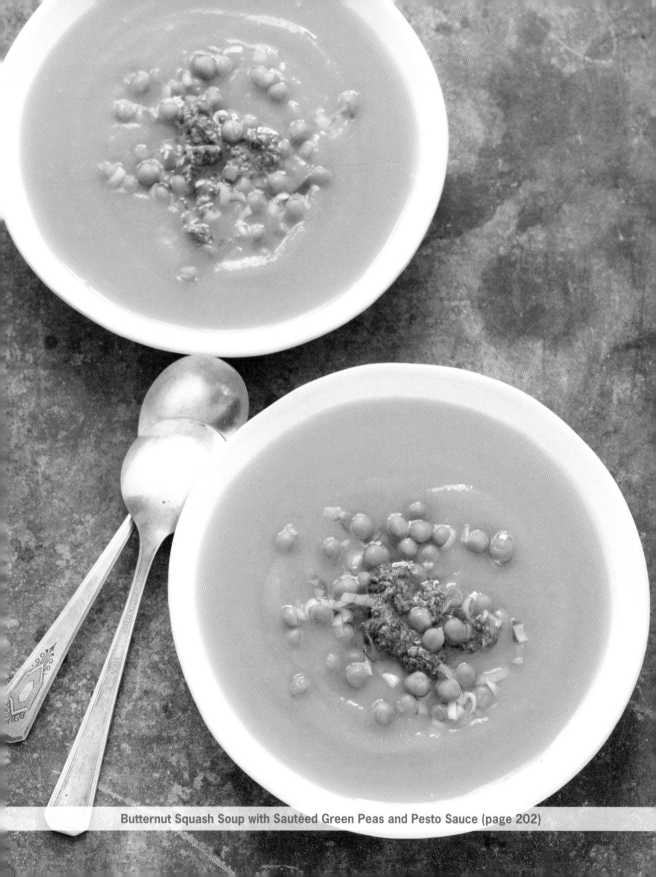

Butternut Squash Soup with Sautéed Green Peas and Pesto Sauce (page 202)

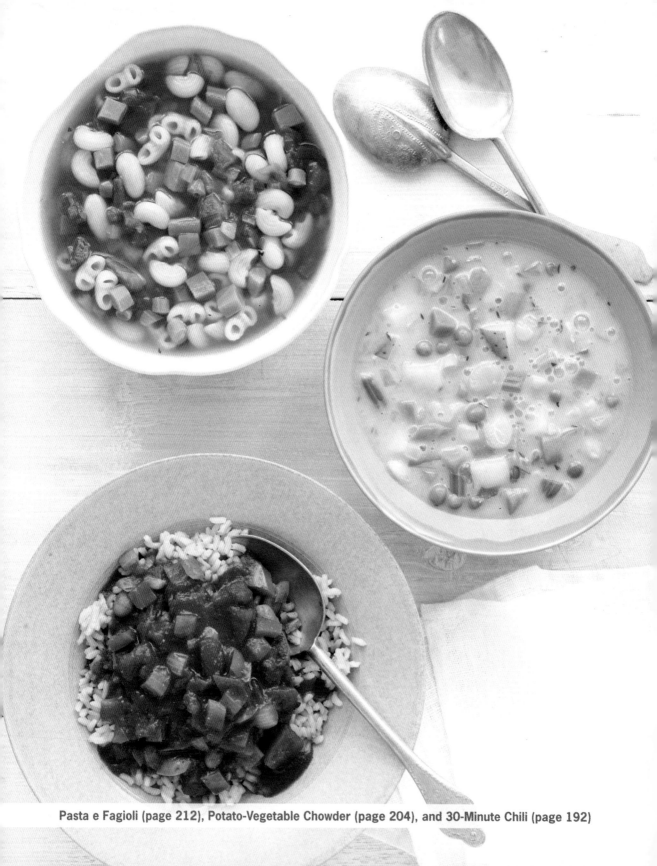

Pasta e Fagioli (page 212), Potato-Vegetable Chowder (page 204), and 30-Minute Chili (page 192)

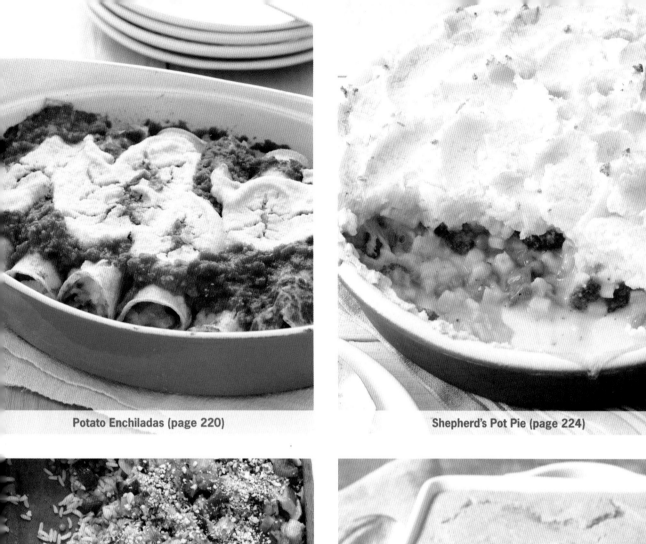

Potato Enchiladas (page 220)

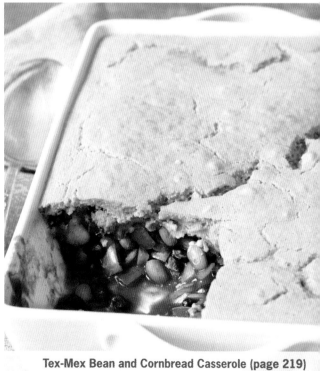

Shepherd's Pot Pie (page 224)

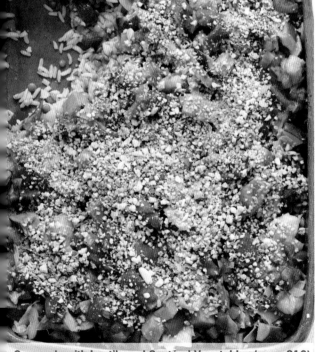

e Casserole with Lentils and Sautéed Vegetables (page 216)

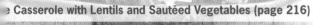

Tex-Mex Bean and Cornbread Casserole (page 219)

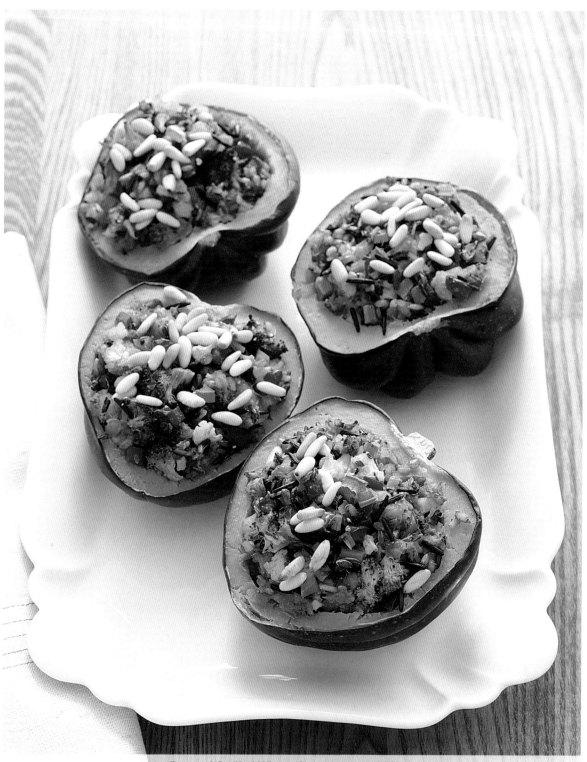

Roasted Stuffed Winter Squash (page 230)

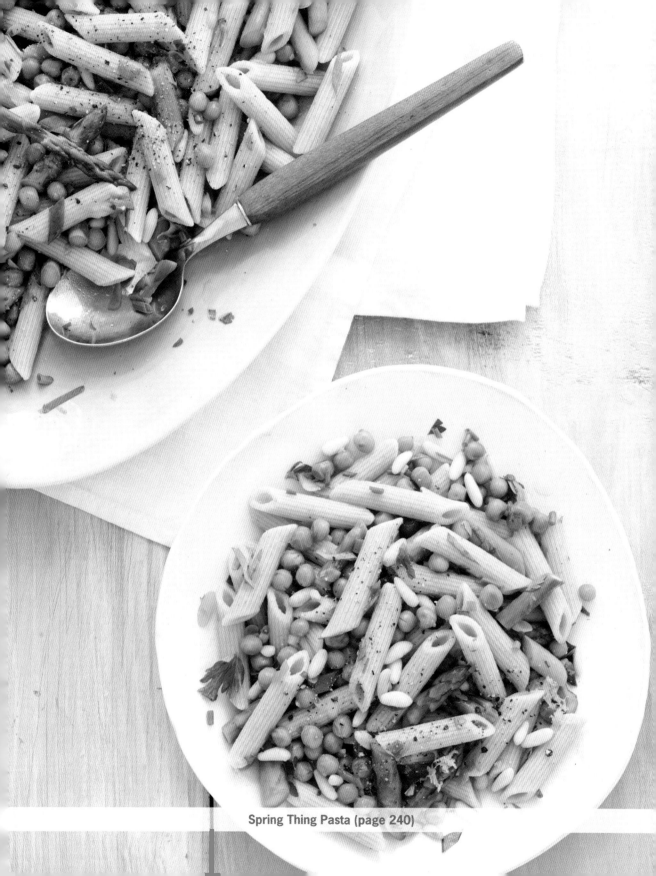

Spring Thing Pasta (page 240)

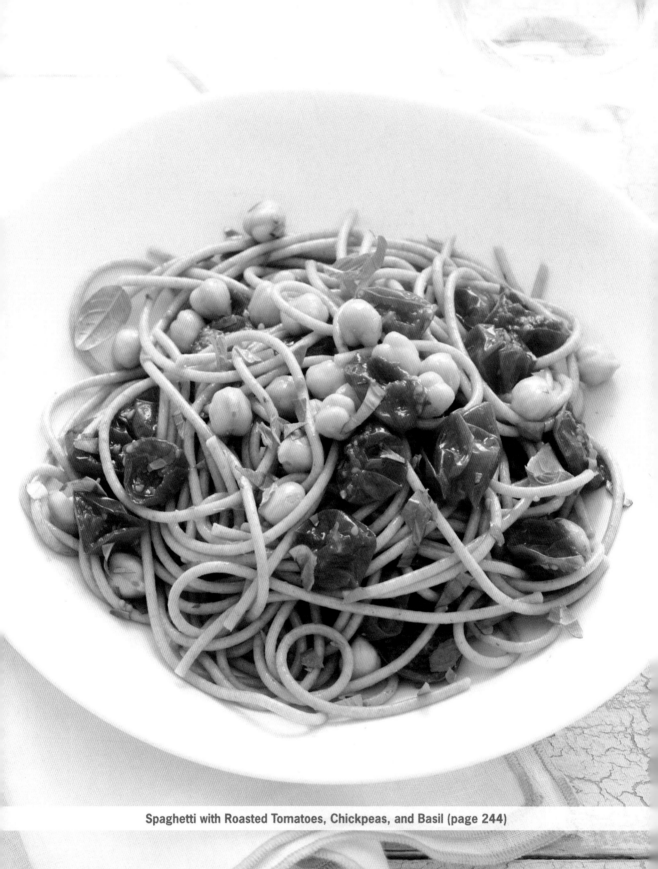

Spaghetti with Roasted Tomatoes, Chickpeas, and Basil (page 244)

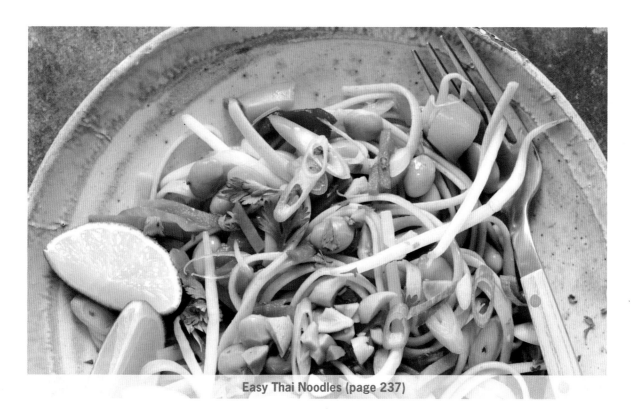

Easy Thai Noodles (page 237)

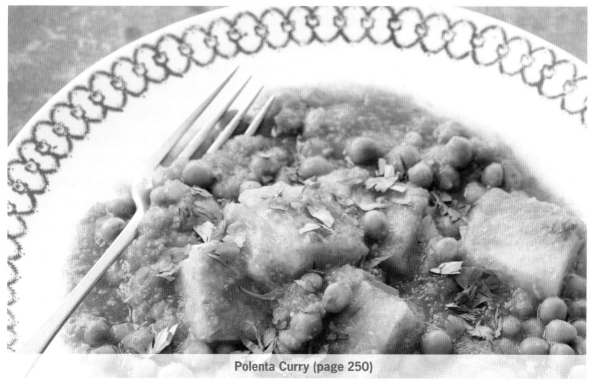

Polenta Curry (page 250)

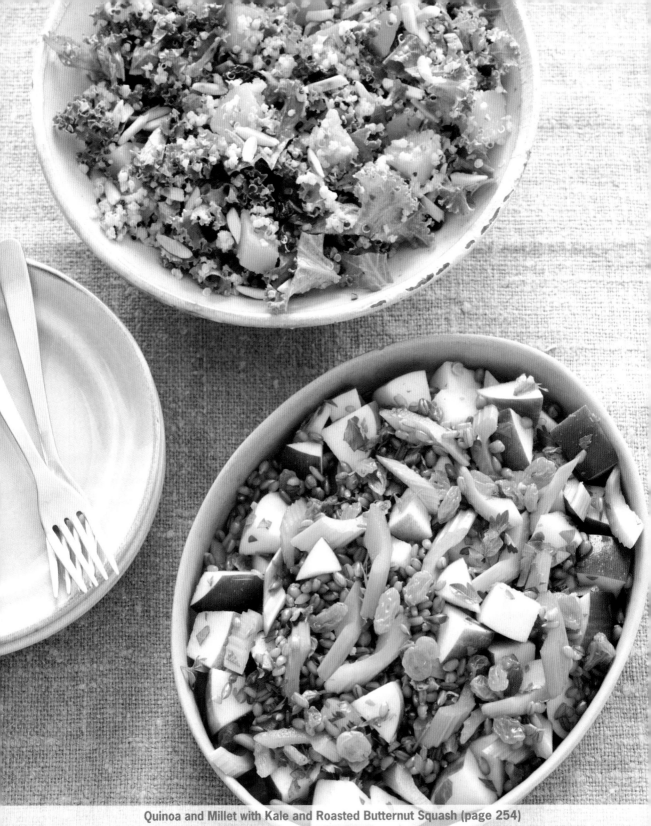

Quinoa and Millet with Kale and Roasted Butternut Squash (page 254)
and Rye and Wheat Berries with Celery and Apples (page 252)

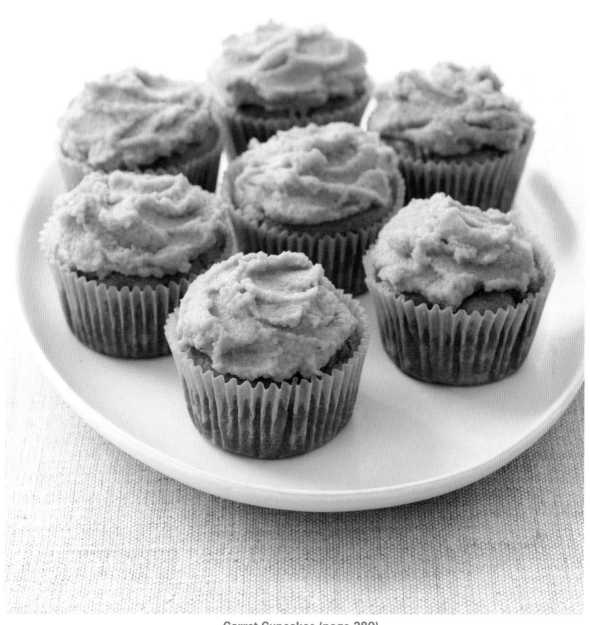

Carrot Cupcakes (page 280)

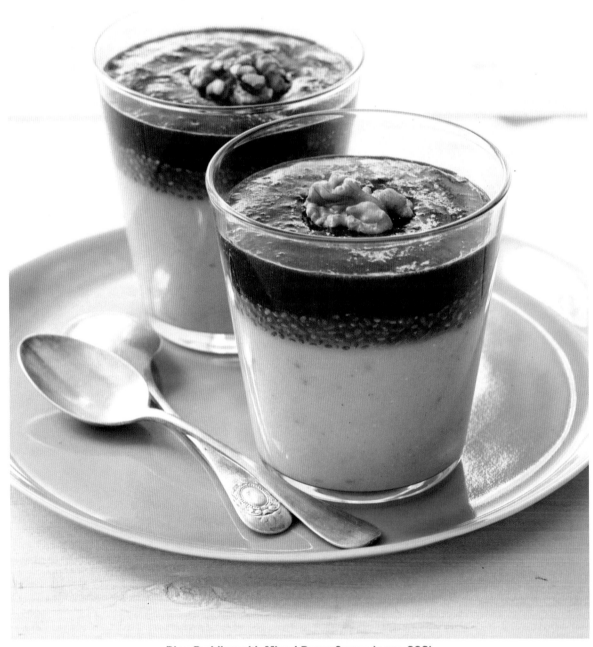

Rice Pudding with Mixed Berry Sauce (page 282)

LET'S GET PRACTICAL:
MAINTAINING A HEALTHY DIET OUTSIDE OF YOUR HOME

There's no getting around it: No matter how simple it is to maintain your healthy diet when you have complete control over the menu, the world outside your door is not always easy to navigate while staying true to your whole-food, plant-based lifestyle. Eating out and traveling can be intimidating, especially in the early months of your transition. And no matter how accommodating the restaurant or your fellow diners, it can feel isolating to be singled out because of your efforts to eat healthier. But these feelings are easily mitigated when you are proactive and prepared.

Eating in Restaurants

First, when eating out with a group, you should try to actively participate in choosing the restaurant. With time, you'll get to know places near you that either have suitable items on their regular menu, or that are happy to accommodate your requests. When traveling, due diligence is key: Before you go, research some good possibilities at your destination. Don't be afraid to call a restaurant in advance and tell them what you're looking for. How welcoming they are to your inquiries by phone can convey all you need to know about how successful and satisfying a meal there would be. Once you know what the good options for restaurants are, you can suggest two or three of them and let your fellow diners pick, confident that wherever you end up there's little risk you'll be hungry when you leave. If you feel like you might not have enough options when you get wherever you're going, you can always eat some healthy food at home before you go. This way you won't be so hungry when you arrive, and you won't be completely dependent on the kitchen to serve you enough.

Of course, it's not always possible to plan ahead of a potential meal out, so there are some practical things you can do when you find yourself in a restaurant that may not obviously cater to your preferred food choices. First and foremost, don't be afraid to ask for clarification of ingredients on the menu. Engage the waitstaff, explain your dietary needs, and help them figure out a way to serve you. (Even make fun of yourself for doing so, just to lighten the mood!) You may suggest, for example, that a dish that's ordinarily pan-fried can instead be steamed or cooked in a bit of vegetable broth or water. Baked potatoes can be served with a bunch of mixed vegetables and without the cheese, butter, and sour cream with which they are often paired. Beans and warm corn tortillas are another example of sides that can easily make a full meal. Do be aware, though, that many common dishes toward which you might gravitate can have hidden ingredients that you wouldn't want to eat. For instance:

- Butter on rice and breads

- Chicken or other animal-based broth in vegetable soups and stews

- Rice cooked in chicken broth

- Bread or pasta made with eggs

- Pork or lard in beans

- Oil in sauces, salsas, and soups

In our experience there are certain types of establishments that are better than others at accommodating us. **Stores and restaurants that bill themselves as "health food" destinations** can be great options, but be aware that even these places tend to lean heavily on oil. Ask them to omit it, and if they seem stumped, suggest that they cook your meal using alternatives that they probably have on hand, such as vegetable broth, black bean sauce, garlic sauce, low-sodium tamari or soy sauce, diced tomatoes, or vinegar.

Salad bars would seem to be an obvious choice, and that can certainly be true, but there are some potential pitfalls here. Remember that not everything in a salad bar is healthy or free of oil- or mayonnaise-based sauces. Stick with whole vegetable toppings and put oil-free dressings on the side. Or bypass the ready-made dressings altogether and use vinegar, or ask for an orange cut in half crosswise and squeeze the juice over your salad for a delicious dressing. Also keep in mind that while dried fruit, nuts, and seeds might be among the healthiest whole foods on the salad bar, they are also very calorie dense, so use them sparingly. Finally, remember that a salad bar is rarely a good source for sufficient healthy calories (unless it includes whole grains or beans), so see if you can order something more filling to go along with the salad, like a baked potato or two.

We've found that at many **ethnic restaurants** it's easy to find delicious food that fits our dietary preferences with very little adjustment. Asian, Italian, and Mexican restaurants, in particular, all tend to have menu standbys like soups that work well as bases for a full meal, especially when you add steamed rice and a big bowl of steamed vegetables. Just make sure you call ahead to check on the common exceptions that we mention in each case below.

Chinese, Vietnamese, Thai, Japanese, and other Asian restaurants have many menu standards that are excellent choices for a whole-food, plant-based eater. Among the appetizers, steamed vegetable dumplings or spring rolls and edamame are good options. Ask for entrées like vegetarian pad thai to be made without oil and eggs. Many vegetarian sushi options are excellent choices. Get a big dish of steamed or boiled rice noodles or plain rice with any combination of vegetables in an oil-free sauce. Feel free to eat white rice if brown rice isn't available; it won't be a problem once in a while. You can use side sauces such as soy sauce, hot sauce, mustard sauce, duck sauce, and so on, either individually or mixed together, to make your own tasty concoction at the table. One thing to look out for at Asian restaurants is that many use fish stock as the standard in every dish that has broth—that means every soup, naturally, but can also apply to sauces and even the poaching or steaming liquid for vegetables. Also confirm that the dumpling wrappers and noodles don't contain eggs.

The kitchens of **Italian restaurants** are usually abundantly stocked with vegetables. Many have vegetable antipasto on their appetizer menus, and of course you can always request a pizza or pasta with tomato sauce and lots of vegetables (hold the cheese, please). Make sure their pasta isn't made with eggs and that their vegetable soups are made with vegetable broth. Also note that more and more Italian restaurants have whole-grain pasta in their kitchens, even if they don't necessarily advertise it on the menu. Ask if this is the case where you're eating, but if all they have is white wheat pasta, don't sweat it as a once-in-a-while option.

Mexican restaurants are great because their staple dish of beans is among our staples, too—just confirm that the rice they serve you is not made with oil and that the beans are made without lard or other pork products. In fact, it's a good idea to call ahead to make sure that not *every* bean dish they serve contains lard, which, in our experience, is sometimes the case. Salsa is always a great choice, and you can bypass the fried chips by asking for soft corn tortillas instead. Entrées such as bean burritos, rice and beans, soft corn tortilla tacos, and grilled vegetable fajitas are all foods we eat at home—it's just really nice to have someone else make them for us now and then!

Of course it can be more challenging when you're on the road and—either because of time or circumstances—your only options are essentially fast-food joints. Here are our solutions to a few common on-the-road scenarios:

- At a **diner**, there's oatmeal, toast, salad, or a baked potato with salsa.

- At a **pizza place**, order a cheese-free pizza with tomato sauce and lots of vegetables.

- At a **sandwich shop**, go for whole-grain bread filled with oil-free vegetables and an oil-free dressing, hummus, or mustard.

We know that this might look like an awful lot to remember, but the best thing about this lifestyle is that with time it becomes second nature. You might want to refer to these suggestions more than once during the early days, but

Traveling Out of Town

When it comes to eating and travel, a little advance planning is all it takes to stay on track. For starters, when we're flying, we bring our own food to eat on the plane. We like to bring a container of hummus (freeze it before you leave to get through security more easily) with chips, carrot sticks, or cooked potato slices for dipping. Dried fruit, such as raisins in small boxes, is very tasty and so convenient for traveling. Fresh fruit is great on planes because it's hydrating and is easily eaten out of hand. Good options are berries, peeled oranges, and apple slices. Or, once we're through security, we'll head to a Mexican or other restaurant that offers baked potatoes and pick up a few for the trip.

When we stay in hotels, eating is easier as long as we ensure that we have a refrigerator and microwave in our room. Then we can bring food with us (which is even easier if we're driving, of course) or buy a selection of in-room foods that will get us through any trip without worrying that we'll be hungry. Here's our go-to list of hotel room foods:

- Oatmeal with fruit or trail mix

- Fresh and/or dried fruit

- Sweet potatoes and/or cut-up mixed vegetables and oil-free dip

- Oil-free chips and salsa

- Whole-grain bread, crackers, or pretzels and dips or nut butter

- Whole-grain cereal and nondairy milk (easy to bring along in a Tupperware and eat)

- Dried or boxed soups (Dr. McDougall makes a brand that is oil-free and low in sodium)

before long you'll be completely in charge of your own diet in such a way that—no matter where you are—you'll know precisely what to look for and what questions to ask.

Eating in Friends' Homes

While we all hope our friends and family will be open to and accepting of our food choices, it can still be uncomfortable for you to ask them to prepare special food just for you. We always offer to bring a dish or two, and we usually make at least one dessert, so there's no risk of our feeling deprived at the end of the meal. Over the years we've found that this approach has two big benefits. First, it removes from our hosts the burden of ensuring we have something to eat, and it allows all of us to simply enjoy each other's company. Second, whatever we bring, we share, and more often than not our hosts and fellow guests enjoy those dishes enormously. This is a wonderful way to demonstrate without preaching that our lifestyle is about good health *and* pleasure—not just the former. There's no better way to relay the message to people than by feeding it to them! And remember, your need for acceptance by your friends and family is real; be sure to take these few small steps so that this need, too, can easily be accomplished without sacrificing your need for health.

EYE ON NUTRITION: CARBOHYDRATES

Plants produce carbohydrates via photosynthesis, the process that uses carbon dioxide and water to convert light energy, i.e., sunlight, into chemical energy stored as glucose. Simple carbohydrates—glucose or fructose—have one or two sugar molecules, while complex carbohydrates have more than two sugar molecules hooked together and include starch (the storage form of carbohydrates in plants) and dietary fiber. But whether a carbohydrate is simple or complex is not where our focus should be when it comes to what we eat. The carbohydrates predominant in fruits, for instance, are simple carbs, but you'll never hear us advising you to avoid those. Remember, it's all about the package. The carbs in highly refined food packages will create health problems. Whole-food, plant-based packages, on the other hand—those found in fruits, vegetables, tubers, whole grains, and legumes—are the very foundation of the Forks Over Knives diet and will lead to good health.

Debunking the "Carbs Are Bad" Myth

Are you coming to this book inclined to believe that carbs cause diabetes and make us fat? If so, you must unlearn everything you think you know about carbohydrates. If you eat a whole-food, plant-based diet, **75 to 80 percent of your calories will come from carbohydrates**—and that is precisely what you want. You don't need to "shoot for" this number; it'll happen naturally, provided your diet is based on fruits, vegetables, tubers, whole grains, and legumes. And let us put your mind at ease: The unrefined carbohydrates in whole or minimally processed plant foods do *not* cause diabetes or make us fat.

Studies show that the lowest rates of diabetes *in the world* are found among populations that consume the *most* carbohydrates.[64] Furthermore, the *Journal of Nutrition* concluded that the data does not support a correlation between high-carbohydrate diets and insulin sensitivity, and an article in *Diabetes Care* concluded that the "Intake of sugars does *not* appear to play a deleterious role in primary prevention of type 2 diabetes" [emphasis added].[65] In fact, the "high-carb" diet that we are recommending—and *not* avoiding carbs—is the exact diet that has *reversed* type 2 diabetes in so many patients.

As for whether carbohydrates make us fat, studies show an inverse association between the consumption of whole grains and weight gain, likely because low-fat, high-carb diets—when those carbs are unrefined—increase satiety and decrease caloric intake. This is because of what we refer to as the "fat-sugar seesaw": When you eat fewer whole carbs (the sugar side of the seesaw), you will inevitably eat more fat. You can subvert this pattern by increasing the whole, minimally processed, unrefined carbs in your diet. By doing so, you will eat less fat.[66] The *American Journal of Clinical Nutrition* said it clearly: "Alter-

THE FORKS OVER KNIVES PLAN

ing the composition of the diet in favor of a higher carbohydrate-to-fat ratio may decrease the incidence of obesity."[67]

The cause of America's obesity epidemic is not whole, unrefined carbohydrates. In fact, carbs are our best energy source because our bodies have evolved to metabolize them very efficiently.[68] Carbs have been shown to be the preferred energy source for athletes.[69] Carbohydrates are also the *primary* source of energy for our brain and the *only* fuel for red blood cells and certain kidney cells.[70] Whole, unrefined, natural carbohydrate-based plant foods also contain dietary fiber (which animal-based and processed foods do not). Dietary fiber satisfies the hunger drive and binds to and assists in the elimination of excess hormones, toxins, cholesterol, and other undesirable matter, and promotes proper bowel function. Fiber also helps to stabilize blood sugar.[71]

Finally, although the predominant macronutrient in whole, plant-based foods is carbohydrates, the package also provides protein (including all of the essential amino acids), essential fatty acids, vitamins, and minerals—all of which are present in healthy amounts; that is, these foods contain neither too little nor too much of these essential nutrients based on our needs.

What *Really* Makes Us Fat?

The major culprit in making us fat is . . . fat. While fat is effortlessly stored on your body, we are very inefficient at converting carbohydrates to fat, a process known as *de novo lipogenesis*.[72] This innate inefficiency means that we must burn significantly more energy—calories—to convert carbohydrates into fat. Plus, fat has more calories per bite of food and thus takes up less space in our stomach. This means we're more likely to overeat when we eat foods higher in fat, as opposed to when we eat foods higher in carbohydrates, which have the bulk to fill us up.

But oftentimes what people think of as a carbohydrate-dominant dish isn't so at all; in fact, it's a high-*fat* dish. Consider the case of the French fry. A baked potato is 87.9 percent carbohydrates, 10.8 percent protein, and 1.2 percent fat—a healthy ratio. Slice that potato and fry it in vegetable oil, however,

What About the Glycemic Index?

We prefer not to talk about the glycemic index because, like other arbitrary health indices, it is a measure of something that has nothing to do with good health. However, misinformation about its alleged importance is pervasive, so we want to clarify what the glycemic index is—and why you don't need to worry about it.

Glycemic Index (GI) measures the rise in blood sugar a person experiences over the two to three hours following the consumption of food that contains 50 grams of carbohydrates and compares this to a standard reference, i.e., the rise in blood sugar when consuming 50 grams of carbohydrates via glucose or white bread. The thought is that you want the GI to be a lower number than pure sugar. But the GI of a food is simply one isolated parameter by which to measure food, and it's a capricious one at that, for it varies with cooking, cooling, or ripening. Furthermore, mixing foods together changes the GI of the meal, but not in a way that can be predicted by knowing each individual food's GI.

Conventional wisdom says a low GI number is good. However, a low GI rating for a food is *not* an indication that it is a *healthy* food. As you increase fat and protein, you decrease a food's GI number because you decrease carbohydrates. Thus chocolate (40) has a lower GI than vegetable soup (48); French fries (63) have a lower GI than boiled potatoes (78); and ice cream (51) has a lower GI than boiled brown rice (68). But sometimes foods with a higher GI—like potatoes and rice—actually better satisfy your appetite and help you avoid overeating. In short, focusing on the Glycemic Index is just as misguided as fixating on individual nutrients. In both cases, hitting a magic "good" number is no indication that the food itself is actually good for you. As we've said before: Focus on the package.

and the change in the macronutrient profile is profound: 53.1 percent carbs, 4.4 percent protein, and 42.5 percent fat. Similarly, consider a bowl of pasta with extra-virgin olive oil—some might consider this the poster child for a high-carb meal. But 4 ounces of whole-grain pasta is 79.3 percent carbohydrates, 14.0 percent protein, and 6.8 percent fat. Add a couple of tablespoons of extra-virgin olive oil to that pasta and the percentage of macronutrients in this "high-carb" dish is 49.9 percent carbohydrate, 8.8 percent protein, and 41.3 percent fat.[73]

These are big differences! The addition of a relatively small volume of pure fat—oil—transforms what appears to be a "plate of carbs" into a food that is fatty and unhealthy.

Remember—you can only eat so much food in a day. If you fill up on carb-based whole foods, you'll push out the refined carbs and fat. Some patients have lost weight and reversed disease simply by adding a baked potato or two before every meal.

The Story on Sugar and How to Embrace Your Sweet Tooth

We are bombarded by stories in the media about how sugar is bad for our health and sweets of all kind should be avoided. However, the desire for sweet-tasting foods is perfectly normal and natural! Indeed, our tongue contains an abundance of sweet receptors for a good reason. Fresh fruit, the source of natural sweetness, is health promoting and an excellent source of calories for the human body. This is why we recommend you include generous amounts of fresh fruit in your diet, and know that it's even okay to make a meal out of nature's candy. If you have never tried this, you may be surprised by just how satisfying it is.

In drawing us to fruit, our sweet tooth was designed to support our long-term health; however, food companies, in an effort to make their products more desirable, use this natural affinity for sweets in a way that brings harm to us. While the simple sugars from whole fruit support human health, the *refined,* or extracted, sugars do not. The refining process removes the water, fiber, and virtually every other nutrient and element of the food. What's left behind is sugar and only sugar—not the package it belongs in. This extraction is more calorie dense and thus overstimulating to our pleasure senses. (Recall that in Week Two we discussed how calorie-dense, concentrated foods lead to excess dopamine being released, resulting in a "high" feeling.) Even worse, food manufacturers add these highly concentrated, palate-pleasing sugars to already stimulating and disease-causing high-fat foods.

There's a point in all this that's not frequently made in the media or by health professionals: Sugar as it occurs in whole foods is not an issue; in fact, it is necessary and should be embraced. It's a problem only when it is extracted from its natural package and used to excess. Also the foods highest in added sugars frequently are higher in added fats, sodium, refined flours, and animal products, making them unhealthy for a variety of reasons and not just because of the added sugars. We hasten to add that even small amounts of added sugars, especially in food made at home, can be enjoyed without posing any significant health risk. That said, desserts and other foods that contain added sugar should be eaten only occasionally and should not be a significant part of your diet. When used on occasion, a small amount of added sugars will contribute only minimal calories to the overall calorie intake in a day, and thus you should not worry about it.

The Takeaway: Carbohydrates

Whole-food carbohydrates neither lead us to diabetes nor make us fat. In fact, your organs prefer carbs to all other nutrients for metabolizing energy, and they are the main fuel for your body and brain. And there is *no other way* to get the healthy fiber you need. Whole, minimally processed, unrefined, plant-based food—in other words, carbohydrate-rich foods—will lead us to optimum health.

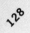

What About Alcohol?

It's been reported in the media and many people think that drinking some alcohol is protective against heart attacks and strokes. There does seem to be a beneficial association between some study populations who moderately drink and their risk of heart disease. However, this relationship is not clearly causal in nature. Furthermore, it turns out that only in the unhealthiest populations does the possibility of such a benefit even exist.

An interesting study looked at "healthy" people and found that there were no longer any cardioprotective effects of alcohol in that population.[74] We are putting "healthy" in quotation marks because we don't know whether this study's definition of healthy was adequate: it was composed of exercising moderately or vigorously a minimum of three hours a week and not smoking, but the published results referenced eating an unspecified amount of fruits and vegetables each day. (It is unclear in the study whether eating as little as a single serving of one or the other each day may have qualified as sufficient.) Yet these habits alone were healthy enough to cancel out any possible benefits of alcohol. The diet recommended in this book is at least as healthy as the diet component in this study. Furthermore, a plant-based diet protects your heart and blood vessels, likely negating any potential positive effect of the alcohol and leaving only the harmful effects.

Alcohol seems to increase the risk of many other problems, including getting cancer (even with very light drinking),[75] cancer recurrence,[76] weight gain,[77] liver damage,[78] and heart arrhythmias.[79] And the more overweight you are, the more likely you are to succumb to liver cancer because obesity and alcohol synergistically increase the risk of incident liver cancer.[80]

In short, there is nothing health-promoting about alcohol. If you do not presently drink alcohol, we urge you not to begin.

That being said, the most important thing you can do for your health is to change your diet over to whole, plant-based foods. So focus on what's easiest for you to change right now. However, if you feel ready to push further toward optimum health, then by all means cut out the alcohol.

MAKING IT WORK FOR YOU:
ADDRESSING SOCIAL PRESSURES

By four weeks into your transition, you've no doubt already had a number of conversations with people about your diet and lifestyle choice, and it's possible that you found some of these encounters uncomfortable. You meet all sorts of different personalities in life, and by extension you'll encounter different perspectives and opinions on your lifestyle choices (come to think of it, when isn't that true?). Reactions can run the gamut from curious to defiant. There are those who will criticize or resist your choice, even if you're doing nothing more than stating what you eat. Among this group might be professionals who believe they *know* that you're causing yourself damage (your own doctor may fall into this category, we're sorry to say). At the other end are those who are truly curious and want to know more. We find that most people fall somewhere between complete rejection and welcoming acceptance. Some might be convinced that they've done exactly what you're doing and it didn't work for them, while others might see the value in what you are doing but are determined that they could "never" live as you are living. It might sometimes seem like the whole world feels entitled to weigh in on a decision that you consider quite personal.

There's no hard-and-fast way to deal with every person you meet who asks you about your diet. It's up to you to address people in a way that's most comfortable for you personally. Sometimes, especially at the beginning of your journey, it's enough simply to understand what sort of encounter you're facing, so you can decide whether to engage kindly or gracefully deflect. Before your transition, it's possible that meeting someone new or seeing someone you hadn't seen in some time wasn't cause for anxiety. But now, when you meet someone for the first time—or the first time in a while—you might suddenly find yourself at the receiving end of what can feel like a torrent of questions:

- Where do you get your protein?

- How do you get enough calcium?

- What about your essential fatty acids?

- Don't potatoes make you fat?

- How on earth do you cook without oil?

- What do you *eat*?

When these questions begin to feel more like an inquisition than a conversation, it's natural to feel a little defensive. So before any conversation can get to the inquisition level, employ a few simple strategies to keep it light. This is pretty easy, actually, because all you need to remember is *why* you are doing what you are doing. Keeping your motives in mind increases your confidence and allows you to address any question from a place of enhanced and quiet confidence.

Don't feel obligated to answer every question that is put to you. Instead, feel free to ask a question or two of your own. For instance, we've found the best response to any of the "Do you get enough [fill in the nutrient here]?" questions is to inquire whether anyone really knows what "enough" means. You've come this far in this book, so *you* know that you don't need to worry about individual nutrients and, furthermore, seeking them can actually be dangerous when the package they come in is damaging to your health in every other way.

You can certainly also acknowledge (with pride!) that you are doing something off the beaten path. You might add something along the lines of "I heard good things about this diet. I tried it and I feel good, so I'm going to stick with it for a while." People who truly care about you should find reassurance in your calm and clear affirmation of your positive state of mind and health. And those who are just trying to pick a fight can't argue with your own assessment of your personal well-being.

It's not complicated: If you sense that someone is asking a good-faith question, you'll likely feel free and happy to share. On the other hand, if you sense that you're talking to someone who is, for whatever reason, seeking only to criticize you, remember that you shouldn't feel compelled to justify your choices. In our experience, no matter what kind of inquiries you're facing, being less forceful and addressing questions in a kind manner is always the way to go.

Rest assured that it does get better over time. As your level of comfort with the lifestyle increases, your confidence with any question will correspondingly increase. Aggressive questioning from other people at this stage can set you back on your heels—that's perfectly normal. But you have made the best possible choice for your health. Trust that you'll eventually find your own sweet spot for answering all sorts of inquiries.

We want to put in a last word about the power of finding a community of like-minded people with whom you can spend time. We *are* out here. Just think about how wonderful it will be when you have compatible partners to eat out with; to travel with; to hike, run, or bike with; and to mutually motivate and support one another. This is not some unreachable Shangri-la. It's within your grasp. The fourth week of your Forks Over Knives lifestyle has arrived. At the end of this week, you get to look forward to the rest of your extraordinary whole-food, plant-based life!*

---

* See page 291 for a handy four-week transition meal planner.

GETTING PERSONAL

Eating is such an uncomplicated joy now. I call this my "piles of food" diet. I can sit down to a huge plate of vegetables, rice, and beans and just eat to my heart's content without feeling gross afterward and without the scale moving up at all.

—Naomi Ninneman, 39, health educator, Cranston, RI

We were formerly on the Paleo diet—so we *loved* adding back in our healthy *carbs*! Guess our bodies needed that. Food is simpler to cook, and things don't have the potential of rotting without proper refrigeration as with meats.

—Amy Denson, 46, homemaker, Lincoln, CA

It is getting so much easier over time. I am now bold enough when we dine out to tell the waiter that I want my veggies water-sautéed. Ha! I had a chef yell in the kitchen about my request (that could be heard in the dining room). He said he had never heard of such a thing. It was hilarious. Well, that chef *did* water-sauté my veggies, and he learned something in the process.

—Jeanne Friedman, 49, retired public school teacher, wellness coach-in-training, Anchorage, AK

When I struggled the most was when I was out with friends for dinner and everyone was eating meat and fried, cheesy food and I was getting the rice pilaf with steamed veggies, and they would say, "Come on, let loose." I stayed motivated to stick with it because I knew I was going to wake up energetic and happy the next day and not with a huge food hangover.

—Cindy Johnson, 35, dental hygienist, Spokane Valley, WA

Going to friends' houses for dinner is hard, but the more people know, it seems most are willing to help and offer to make something you can eat, or learn not to be offended when I bring my own food. Also, the longer I've been eating whole-food, plant-based, the less tempting other food is, so it really doesn't bother me much! I just make sure I always carry something with me, like pumpkin seeds and raisins or something to hold me over.

—Jill Pierce, 31, health and fitness coach and stay-at-home mom, Carver, MA

I would visit home and my mom would make a lot of my favorite dishes that I no longer desired (she sometimes forgets that I do not eat dairy or eggs). It was hard to turn down these items and disappoint her, but over time she has embraced a plant-based diet as well. Way to go, Mom!

—Cole Adam, 26, registered dietician, Denver, CO

I decided to watch *Forks Over Knives* every 6 to 12 months as a refresher. There is no "one and done."

—Liz Goode, 65, software tech support, retired attorney, New York, NY

I've gone to potlucks to meet other people who do the same thing. It helps if you're not the only person you know doing this. I menu plan every week and have things planned out so that I'm never worried about what I'll eat. I am actually enjoying food now and I just see this getting better and better. . . . As an added bonus, I've watched my teenage son thrive after making this change as well. I'm so grateful we both made this change. Plant strong for life!

—Janet Beckman, 42, accounting, Tualatin, OR

CONCLUSION:
You're on Your Way!

Congratulations on making it through your four-week transition! You have made an impressive and critical change in your life, and this is reason to really cheer. We hope you are seeing results and will achieve all that you set out to accomplish a month ago. This is the beginning of an exciting and worthwhile journey.

Just like all journeys, there will almost certainly be bumps in the road. There may be a time when you are drawn to the unhealthy foods that you've let go of over the past month. The key is to be prepared when you hit those bumps. There's no need to vow that you will *never* do something again—like saying that you'll never have another chicken sandwich or chocolate milkshake. We suggest something simpler: Promise yourself that if you begin to feel strong cravings for unhealthy foods, you'll pause long enough to contemplate what it is you're really missing.

Taking the time to reflect can keep you motivated and on course toward reaching your goals. During a challenging time, it could be very helpful to reread parts, or all, of this book. Remember the basics and ensure that your lifestyle meets your needs for health, ease, pleasure, and acceptance (see page 40). Upon reflection, you might remind yourself how to plan satisfying meals (see page 79); how to cope with the difficulties that you may face when

THE FORKS OVER KNIVES PLAN

traveling (see page 121); or how to get along with people who eat differently (see page 129). Holding off on poor food choices gives you time to understand the big picture, so that your decisions are governed by thoughtful consideration rather than the emotions of the moment.

Dr. Caldwell B. Esselstyn, Jr., one of the experts featured in *Forks Over Knives,* likes to say that people choosing a whole-food, plant-based lifestyle become "the locus of control" of their own health and vitality. We couldn't agree more. Our favorite thing about the lifestyle is seeing how our patients, friends, and family become empowered. They no longer feel helpless or at the mercy of the health care system. We want this for you, too. We want you to be active through your golden years, playing with your grandchildren, dancing, hiking, gardening, enjoying a night out, or contributing to your community in whatever way brings you contentment. It may sound clichéd, but the power is in your hands. In this food-over-medicine way of life, we may provide the information, but *you* hold the prescription pad.

Thank you for allowing us to share our knowledge and experience with you. Good luck as you journey on. And one last thing: Don't forget to eat your potato enchiladas!

PART III

THE RECIPES

It is much easier to keep our kitchen clean. Cooking meat and cheese makes a mess that is hard to scour off pots, oven walls, and the range hood.

—Richard Hamje, 57, IT consultant, Portland, OR

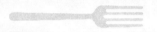

Cooking without oil was initially a challenge but really much easier than expected. Explaining to friends why we are not using "heart–healthy" oils has been hard. People do not want to think poorly of olive oil.

—Sue Rose, 63, retired, Rochester, NY

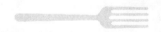

Once you start to make the changes, fried fatty foods and meat seriously do not taste good. I just cannot eat how I used to because I do not like it anymore.

—Suzi Fenn, 49, interior designer, Berkeley, CA

It's no secret that your chances for success with any new endeavor are improved enormously when you have the proper tools. As far as we're concerned, there's no better route to embracing your new lifestyle than enjoying delicious food! To that end we've brought in Forks Over Knives friends Darshana Thacker and Del Sroufe to provide us with some amazing recipes. We are very glad to know both of them personally and have seen firsthand their impressive talent for creating approachable recipes that give delectable results. You'll hear directly from both of them in the following pages, and you'll know which chef you're hearing from by their initials at the end of each recipe's headnote. Before we turn the stage completely over to them, we'll take a moment to introduce you to these wonderful, talented chefs.

Darshana Thacker's best memories are the fun-filled summer holidays spent in her mother's family home in a small town near Mumbai, India. During the summertime, she spent a lot of time in the big kitchen learning how herbs, spices, and foods should be mixed together to create the finest vegetarian homemade dining. In 2001, Darshana migrated to the United States. She adopted a 100 percent plant-based diet that was consistent with her values and best for her health. She feels more energetic, stronger, more creative, and happier than ever before. Today she makes food with the care and precision that she learned from the cooks in her family, but using only whole-food,

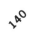

plant-based ingredients. Darshana's recipes have been published in *L.A. Yoga Magazine*, *Forks Over Knives: The Plant-Based Way to Health*, and *Forks Over Knives—The Cookbook*. You'll recognize her recipes going forward by her initials, *DT.*

Del Sroufe's personal story is gripping and will ring familiar to many. He was lucky enough to be born into a family that revered food. However, he was *unlucky* enough that the foods they revered, by and large, were animal-based. Even after Del switched to a vegan diet, he still put on a significant amount of weight, learning firsthand that a vegan diet is not necessarily a *healthy* diet. It was when he turned to a whole-food, plant-based diet that he lost more than 200 pounds! His wonderful cookbook *Better Than Vegan* tells the story of his struggle with weight gain and loss and contains 101 fabulous recipes to boot. Del is also the author of *Forks Over Knives—The Cookbook*, so his approachable, tasty recipes are familiar to many readers worldwide.

Del has been cooking in vegetarian and plant-based kitchens for twenty-five years. He is currently co-owner and chef at Wellness Forum Foods, a meal delivery and catering service based in Columbus, Ohio. He teaches whole-food, plant-based cooking classes and travels the country talking about his own struggles with diet and weight. You'll know him in these pages as *DS.*

BREAKFAST

Multigrain Pancakes with Fresh Berries

Makes about 12 pancakes

You might think it's difficult to get light and fluffy whole-grain pancakes, let alone without adding oil to the batter. I am happy to be the one to tell you that it's actually as easy as making this recipe! —DS

1½ cups whole wheat pastry flour

¼ cup cornmeal or other whole-grain flour

¼ cup rolled oats

1 tablespoon aluminum-free baking powder

½ teaspoon sea salt

¼ teaspoon ground cinnamon

⅛ teaspoon freshly grated nutmeg

1¾ cups unsweetened, unflavored plant milk

½ cup unsweetened applesauce

2 tablespoons pure maple syrup, plus more for serving, if desired

1 cup fresh blueberries, raspberries, or sliced strawberries, for serving

Apple butter, for serving (optional)

1. Preheat the oven to 200°F.
2. In a large bowl, whisk together the flour, cornmeal, oats, baking powder, salt, cinnamon, and nutmeg until well combined. Make a well in the center of the flour mixture and add the plant milk, applesauce, and maple syrup. Gently fold the ingredients together just until incorporated. Do not overmix; the batter will be lumpy.
3. Heat a griddle or large nonstick pan over medium heat until a few droplets of water dropped in the pan jump and sizzle.
4. Spoon ⅓ cup batter for each pancake onto the pan until no more will fit. Cook 3 to 4 minutes until the edges look dry and the bottoms are crisp and lightly browned. Using a spatula, turn the pancakes over and cook for 2 to 3 minutes more. Transfer the pancakes to a heatproof platter and place in the oven to keep warm. Repeat with the remaining batter.
5. Serve the pancakes topped with fruit and a little maple syrup or apple butter.

Corn and Black Bean Cakes

Makes about 10 pancakes

*My mom made a version of these savory pancakes for dinner when
I was a kid. My updated version is healthier, but no less delicious—
and now I enjoy them for breakfast, too. For best results, don't
try to flip the pancakes until they are thoroughly crisped on the
underside; only then will they release from the pan easily. —DS*

1½ cups whole wheat pastry
flour

½ cup cornmeal

1 tablespoon aluminum-free
baking powder

½ teaspoon sea salt

1½ cups unsweetened,
unflavored plant milk

¼ cup unsweetened
applesauce

1 medium red bell pepper,
seeded and finely diced

1 (10-ounce) package frozen
corn kernels, thawed

1 cup cooked or canned black
beans, rinsed and drained

6 green onions, white and light
green parts thinly sliced

Tomato Salsa (page 274,
or use store-bought), for
serving

Sour "Cream" (page 269), for
serving

Chopped fresh cilantro, for
serving

1. Preheat the oven to 200°F.

2. In a large bowl, whisk together the flour,
   cornmeal, baking powder, and salt until well
   combined. Make a well in the center of the flour
   mixture and add the plant milk, applesauce,
   bell pepper, corn, black beans, and green
   onions. Gently fold the ingredients together
   just until incorporated. Do not overmix.

3. Heat a griddle or large nonstick pan over
   medium heat until a few droplets of water
   dropped in the pan jump and sizzle.

4. Spoon ½ cup batter for each pancake onto
   the pan, making sure they don't touch each
   other, until no more will fit. Cook until the
   undersides are crisp and the pancake can be
   flipped easily without falling apart, about
   4 minutes. Using a spatula, turn the pancakes
   over and cook until the other side is lightly
   browned and crisp, about 4 minutes. Transfer

the pancakes to a heatproof platter and place in the oven to keep warm. Repeat with the remaining batter.

5. Serve the pancakes topped with salsa, sour "cream," and chopped cilantro.

RECIPES

THE FORKS OVER KNIVES PLAN

RECIPES

The Easiest Granola
Makes about 4 cups

I think it doesn't occur to many people that you can actually make granola really easily in your own kitchen. Plus, when so many different companies make it, from major cereal producers to tiny companies with cute names, people may wonder why they'd bother since it is so readily available. But store-bought granola is usually made with far more dried fruit and nuts than I want—not to mention added oil. I prefer to have control over what goes into my granola, and then I'm free to embellish it the way I want to—perhaps sprinkled on top of a big bowl of fresh fruit one day and topped with a small handful of nuts or dried fruit and a bit of plant milk on another. And when it's as easy to pull together as this recipe is (and cheaper than buying it premade), the reasons to make it myself far outweigh whatever reasons there might be to buy it. —DS

¼ cup peanut butter or other nut butter

¼ cup pure maple syrup

1 teaspoon pure vanilla extract

¼ teaspoon sea salt

4 cups rolled oats

1. Preheat the oven to 300°F. Line a large baking sheet with parchment paper.
2. Place the peanut butter, maple syrup, vanilla, sea salt, and ½ cup water in a blender. Process until smooth and creamy.
3. Place the oats in a large bowl and pour the peanut butter mixture over them. Mix until the oats are well coated. Spread the mixture evenly over the parchment-lined baking sheet.
4. Bake until the oats are dry to the touch and lightly browned, stirring occasionally, 40 to 50 minutes. Turn the oven off, but leave the granola in the oven until it has cooled completely.
5. Store the granola in an airtight container at room temperature for up to 10 days.

The Quickest Breakfast Wrap

Makes 1 wrap

This no-cook breakfast comes together in a flash and travels well. —DS

1 (10-inch) whole-grain tortilla

2 tablespoons nut butter, such as peanut, almond, or cashew

1 tablespoon unsweetened apple butter or other fruit butter

1 ripe banana, sliced

2 tablespoons raisins

1. Place the tortilla on a flat surface. Spread the nut butter across the middle of the tortilla and top with the apple butter, banana, and raisins.

2. Fold the ends of the tortilla in toward the center, and roll the wrap up like a burrito. Serve.

RECIPES

Twice-Baked Breakfast Sweet Potatoes

Makes 4 sweet potatoes

These are always a hit at winter weekend brunch, although I've often thought they'd be just as nice as a dessert. The aroma of cinnamon and toasted nuts wafts through the house even before you serve them—a tantalizing promise of what's to come. —DS

4 large sweet potatoes, scrubbed

1 (20-ounce) can crushed pineapple in juice, drained well

2 tablespoons pure maple syrup

2 teaspoons ground cinnamon

Sea salt

¼ cup chopped pecans, toasted (see below)

¼ cup grated unsweetened coconut

1. Preheat the oven to 350°F.

2. Place the sweet potatoes on a baking sheet and bake until they are tender when pierced with a sharp knife or a fork, about 1 hour. Remove the sweet potatoes from the oven and let them cool; leave the oven on.

3. When they are cool enough to handle, cut a slit lengthwise down the center of each potato. Scoop out the flesh, leaving a layer about ½ inch thick attached to the skin inside to form a shell. Transfer the flesh to a large bowl and add the pineapple, 1 tablespoon of the maple syrup, the cinnamon, and salt to taste.

4. Stir until well blended. Spoon the filling into the cavity of each potato. Return the potatoes to the baking sheet and set aside.

5. In a small bowl, combine the toasted pecans, coconut, and remaining 1 tablespoon maple syrup and stir until well blended. Spoon the mixture on top of the sweet potato filling,

dividing it evenly among the potatoes. Bake until the coconut is lightly browned, about 25 minutes. Serve.

How to Toast Nuts

Place nuts in a medium skillet and toast over medium-low heat, stirring frequently, until lightly browned and fragrant, 4 to 7 minutes. Watch them carefully so that they don't burn. Immediately transfer the nuts to a plate to stop the cooking and let stand until cool.

Breakfast Smoothie

Makes about 3 cups

Smoothies are great for breakfast because they come together quickly, taste great, and are full of whole-food goodness. Be sure to use bananas that have brown spots on their peels; these are truly ripe and will taste best. Also feel free to use this recipe as a jumping-off point and use whatever fruit you love or have handy. Sometimes I like to add chopped ripe mango along with the berries.—DT

3 ripe bananas, sliced

2 cups frozen or fresh berries

Water or unsweetened, unflavored plant milk as needed

1. Place the bananas and berries in a blender.
2. Process until smooth and creamy, adding water or milk as needed to keep the mixture moving and to achieve the desired consistency. Serve immediately.

Breakfast Fruit Crisp

Makes one (8 × 8-inch) pan

This is a year-round recipe—just change the fruit according to what's available in your produce section, or at the market, or even in your freezer. Fresh or frozen berries of any kind are great, as are diced apples or pears (don't defrost the fruit before using—just toss it in frozen). You can even combine fruits, such as diced pears and blackberries, mixed berries, or peaches and strawberries. And one final, important note: The main difference between the fruit crisp I eat for dessert and the one I eat for breakfast is the time of day I eat it! —DS

FOR THE TOPPING

2 cups rolled oats

½ teaspoon ground cinnamon

¼ teaspoon sea salt

2½ tablespoons pure maple syrup

½ cup unsweetened applesauce

FOR THE FILLING

6 cups fresh or frozen blueberries or other fruit

2 tablespoons pure maple syrup

3 tablespoons arrowroot powder

2 tablespoons fresh lemon juice (from about 1 lemon)

1 teaspoon ground cinnamon

Pinch of sea salt

1. Preheat the oven to 350°F.

2. To make the topping, in a large bowl, whisk together the oats, cinnamon, and salt until well combined. Add the maple syrup and applesauce and use a wooden spoon to stir until well combined. Set aside.

3. To make the filling, in a large bowl, combine the blueberries, maple syrup, arrowroot powder, lemon juice, cinnamon, and salt. Toss gently until well combined.

4. Spoon the filling mixture into an 8-inch square baking dish and scatter the oat topping evenly over the top.

5. Bake for 20 minutes, then reduce the oven temperature to 325°F and bake until the topping is lightly browned, 20 to 25 minutes more.

RECIPES

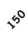

Potato Scramble with Hot Chile Sauce

Makes about 6 cups scramble

This hearty dish is easy to prepare ahead of time, which makes it ideal for holiday breakfasts and a good option to serve for brunch. When you're ready to serve, simply reheat the potatoes and spoon them on top of toast or roll up in tortillas. To make it a bigger meal, serve it with a side of steamed greens or vegetables or with a salad. —DT

1½ cups chopped red onion

3 tablespoons prepared yellow mustard

¼ teaspoon ground allspice

1½ teaspoons finely chopped seeded jalapeño

2 pounds potatoes, any variety, scrubbed and cut into ½-inch cubes

Sea salt

2 ripe medium tomatoes, finely chopped (about 1 cup)

½ cup fresh cilantro, finely chopped

3 tablespoons fresh lime juice (from 1 to 2 limes)

6 slices whole-grain bread, toasted, or 6 whole-grain tortillas, warmed (see page 159)

Hot Chile Sauce (page 272), for serving (optional)

1. In a skillet, combine the onion, mustard, allspice, jalapeño, and 1 cup water. Stir to combine and bring to a simmer over medium heat. Cover the pan and cook until the onions are translucent, 5 to 10 minutes. Add the potatoes, salt to taste, and an additional 1 cup water. Raise the heat to high, cover, and cook, stirring once or twice, for 5 minutes. Reduce the heat to medium and continue to cook, covered, until the potatoes are tender when pierced with a sharp knife, 10 to 15 minutes. You can prepare the dish to this point up to 2 days ahead; just transfer the potato mixture to an airtight container and store in the refrigerator until ready to serve.

2. To serve, reheat over low heat if necessary. Just before serving, stir in the tomatoes, cilantro, and lime juice. Place the bread on plates and top them with the potato scramble. (Alternatively, wrap the scramble in warmed whole-grain tortillas.) If desired, drizzle Hot Chile Sauce over the top or pass it in a bowl at the table.

Big Breakfast Burrito

Makes 4 burritos; about 6 cups filling

When I have a little extra time to make a hearty breakfast, I often make these burritos. For a change of pace, try a couple of medium, red-skinned or Yukon Gold potatoes in place of the sweet potato, and if you have it around, toss in ¼ cup of chopped fresh basil. Yum! —DS

1 medium yellow onion, diced

1 medium red bell pepper, seeded and diced

1 large sweet potato, peeled and finely diced

3 cloves garlic, minced

2 tablespoons dried basil

2 teaspoons ground turmeric

1 teaspoon dried thyme

1 pound extra-firm tofu, crumbled

¼ cup nutritional yeast

Sea salt and freshly ground black pepper

4 large whole-grain tortillas

Tomato Salsa (page 274), for serving

1. Preheat the oven to 350°F.
2. In a large skillet, cook the onion, bell pepper, and sweet potato over medium heat, stirring occasionally and adding water 1 tablespoon at a time as needed to keep the vegetables from sticking, until the sweet potato is tender and the onions start to brown, about 10 minutes.
3. Add the garlic, basil, turmeric, and thyme and cook until the garlic has softened, about 1 minute. Add the tofu and nutritional yeast to the pan and season with salt and black pepper.
4. Spoon the mixture onto a nonstick baking sheet, spreading it evenly. Bake, turning occasionally, until the tofu is lightly browned, about 35 minutes.
5. To serve, place a tortilla on a plate. Spoon one-quarter of the tofu scramble in the center of the tortilla. Spoon some of the salsa over the scramble. Fold the two sides of the tortilla into the center. Starting at the bottom, roll the tortilla up. Repeat with the remaining tortillas, tofu scramble, and salsa. Serve.

Fruit and Nut Oatmeal

Makes about 1½ cups

Oatmeal is one of my favorite breakfast foods. It is quick to prepare and easily adaptable to my ever-changing moods—some days I want it with fruit, some days I want it plain, and sometimes I want a little bit of everything in it (that's when I add all of the add-ons listed here!). This basic recipe is all you need to get started—add as much or as little of the extras as you like. —DS

¾ **cup rolled oats**

¼ **teaspoon ground cinnamon**

Pinch of sea salt

¼ **cup fresh berries (optional)**

½ **ripe banana, sliced (optional)**

2 tablespoons chopped nuts, such as walnuts, pecans, or cashews (optional)

2 tablespoons dried fruit, such as raisins, cranberries, chopped apples, chopped apricots (optional)

Maple syrup (optional)

1. Combine the oats and 1½ cups water in a small saucepan. Bring to a boil over high heat. Reduce the heat to medium-low and cook until the water has been absorbed, about 5 minutes. Stir in the cinnamon and sea salt.

2. Top with the berries, banana, nuts, and/or dried fruit as you like. If desired, pour a little maple syrup on top. Serve hot.

RECIPES

Baked Breakfast Polenta with Berry Compote

Makes about 12 (½-inch-thick) polenta slices and about 2 cups compote

Pretty much any fruit dessert I make lends itself to swapping out whatever fruit I "usually" use for whatever fruit is in season, and therefore most delicious at the time. This recipe is no exception. While any individual berry may only be fully in season for a few weeks, the overall berry season is nice and long, with blueberries, raspberries, strawberries, and blackberries all coming into season at slightly different times. Feel free to use whatever looks and tastes best to you right now! —DS

1 (18-ounce) package precooked polenta, sliced crosswise ½ inch thick

1 quart fresh strawberries, hulled and quartered

2 tablespoons pure maple syrup

1 tablespoon fresh lemon juice

Pinch of sea salt

1. Preheat the oven to 450°F.
2. Place the polenta on a nonstick baking sheet and bake until the polenta is hot, 13 to 15 minutes.
3. While the polenta bakes, in a medium saucepan, combine the strawberries, maple syrup, lemon juice, and salt and cook over medium heat until the berries start to break down, 7 to 8 minutes.
4. Serve the polenta topped with the berry compote.

RECIPES

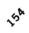

THE FORKS OVER KNIVES PLAN

RECIPES

WRAPS, ROLL-UPS, AND BURGERS

Black-Eyed Pea Burgers

Makes 4 burgers

If you're like me, you're probably tired of the same old black bean burger. Here's a great alternative, made with flavorful, earthy black-eyed peas. —DS

½ cup cornmeal

1 (15-ounce) can black-eyed peas, rinsed and drained

1 small yellow onion, minced

1 stalk celery, minced

1 medium carrot, minced

2 cloves garlic, minced

3 tablespoons arrowroot powder

1 teaspoon ground cumin

Sea salt and freshly ground black pepper

4 whole-grain sandwich buns, for serving (optional)

1 large tomato, sliced, for serving (optional)

Lettuce leaves, for serving (optional)

Mustard and ketchup, for serving (optional)

1. Place the cornmeal on a shallow plate and set aside. Have a nonstick baking sheet ready or line a regular baking sheet with parchment paper.

2. Place the black-eyed peas in a medium bowl. Using a potato masher, smash the peas, leaving some of them intact for texture. Add the onion, celery, carrot, garlic, arrowroot powder, cumin, and salt and pepper to taste. Using a wooden spoon or rubber spatula, mix until well blended; the mixture will be very crumbly.

3. Divide the mixture into four equal portions. Press each portion into a patty about 4 inches across and dredge them in the cornmeal to coat completely. Transfer to the baking sheet and chill for 1 hour.

4. Preheat the oven to 350°F.

5. Remove the burgers from the refrigerator and bake for 20 to 25 minutes. Turn each patty over and bake until the burgers are lightly browned and hold together well when moved, 15 to 20 minutes more.

6. If desired, place each burger on the bottom half of a bun and top with lettuce, tomato, mustard, and ketchup. Top each with the other half of the bun and serve.

RECIPES

THE FORKS OVER KNIVES PLAN

RECIPES

Sloppy Joe Pitas

Makes 6 sloppy joe pitas; about 4 cups filling

*Sloppy joes have always been one of my favorite go-to meals.
They are comfort food at its best, and in a pita, they even travel
far better than the original burger-bun versions! —DS*

1 cup medium-grind bulgur

1 medium onion, finely chopped

½ medium green bell pepper, finely chopped

1 stalk celery, finely chopped

2 cloves garlic, minced

1¾ cups Del's Basic Barbecue Sauce (page 270, or use store-bought)

1 tablespoon low-sodium soy sauce or tamari

Sea salt and freshly ground black pepper

3 whole-grain pita breads

1. In a small saucepan, bring 2 cups water to a boil. Stir in the bulgur. Turn off the heat, cover the pan, and let the bulgur steep while you prepare the rest of the dish, at least 15 minutes.

2. In a large skillet, combine the onion, bell pepper, and celery. Cook over medium heat, stirring occasionally and adding water 1 tablespoon at a time as needed to keep the vegetables from sticking, until the onions start to brown, 7 to 8 minutes. Add the garlic and cook until softened, about 1 minute.

3. Drain the bulgur if necessary and add it to the pan with the onion mixture. Add the barbecue sauce and soy sauce and mix well. Reduce the heat to medium-low and cook, stirring occasionally, until the sauce thickens a little, about 10 minutes. Season to taste with salt and black pepper.

4. Lightly heat the pitas in a toaster or on a dry skillet over medium heat for about 20 seconds per side, making sure they do not get crisp.

5. Cut the pitas in half. Spoon the sloppy joe filling into each of the six pita halves. Serve warm.

6. If you have leftover filling, store it in an airtight container in the refrigerator for up to 4 days.

RECIPES

Black Bean and Rice Burritos

Makes 8 burritos; about 8 cups filling

*This bean and rice burrito is best served warm, but cold leftovers
make a very good packed lunch the next day. —DT*

FOR THE FILLING

1 cup medium-grain brown
   rice, rinsed (see page 243)

1 cup finely chopped onions

2 cloves garlic, minced

1½ teaspoons finely chopped
   seeded jalapeño

2 teaspoons ground cumin

1 tablespoon dried oregano

5 small or 2 to 3 large bay
   leaves

1 cup dried black beans,
   soaked (see page 160)

1 cup diced zucchini

1 cup diced red bell pepper

1½ teaspoons white wine
   vinegar

1 tablespoon fresh lemon juice

Sea salt and ground black
   pepper

FOR THE SALSA

1 cup finely chopped green
   onions, white and light green
   parts

1 cup finely chopped
   tomatoes

½ cup finely chopped fresh
   cilantro

1 tablespoon fresh lemon juice

1. To prepare the filling, in a medium saucepan, combine the rice and 2½ cups water and bring to a boil over high heat. Reduce the heat to low, cover the pan, and simmer for 45 minutes.

2. Meanwhile, in a separate medium saucepan, combine the onions, garlic, jalapeño, cumin, oregano, bay leaves, and 1 cup water. Bring to a boil over medium heat and cook, covered, for 10 minutes. Add the soaked beans to the pot, along with enough water to cover them. Bring to a boil. Cover the pan and cook until the beans are tender, 25 to 45 minutes.

3. Add the zucchini, bell pepper, and vinegar and cook, covered, for 10 minutes more.

4. Add the cooked rice, lemon juice, and salt and pepper to taste, and mix well. Cook, uncovered, until all the liquid has been absorbed. Taste and adjust the seasoning. Remove from the heat, remove the bay leaves, and cover the pan to keep the beans and rice warm until ready to assemble the burritos.

5. To make the salsa, in a small bowl, combine the green onions, tomatoes, cilantro, and

TO ASSEMBLE

2 avocados

1 tablespoon fresh lemon juice

8 large whole-grain tortillas

Hot sauce, for serving
   (optional)

lemon juice. Toss gently to combine. (You'll have about 2½ cups.) Set aside.

6. To serve, cut each avocado in half and remove and discard the pit. Use a thin knife to cut each half lengthwise into thin slices, being careful not to cut through the skin. Use a spoon to gently scoop the sliced avocado out of the skin and into a shallow bowl. Drizzle the avocado slices with the lemon juice. Set aside.

7. Warm the tortillas for about 20 seconds on each side in a dry skillet set over medium heat. Place one warmed tortilla on a plate. Place about ¾ cup of the rice and bean filling in the center of the tortilla and flatten the filling slightly, leaving at least 2 inches of the tortilla uncovered on either side. Top with 1 to 2 tablespoons of the salsa and 3 or 4 slices of avocado.

8. Fold in both sides of the tortilla, and then fold up the bottom to cover the filling. Roll the tortilla away from you while securing the two sides that have been folded in. Place the tortilla seam-side down on a serving platter. Repeat with the remaining tortillas and fillings.

Black Bean and Rice Burritos *(cont.)*

9. These are best served warm, with hot sauce, if desired.
10. If you must wait a little bit before serving, individually wrap each burrito tightly in parchment or waxed paper until ready to serve (you can refrigerate any leftovers in this manner as well). This ensures that they will hold together better when served later.

Soaking and Cooking Beans and Substituting Canned Beans for Dried

Almost all beans and many legumes are best if they are soaked before cooking. It's practically effortless if you think ahead and put them in water the night before or the same morning that you're cooking them. But if you don't think of it in time, there's a very easy quick-soak option.

To soak beans and legumes the traditional way, place them in a bowl and cover generously with water. Set aside to soak for 6 hours or overnight. Drain and cook as directed in the recipe.

For the quick soak, place the beans or legumes in a saucepan and cover generously with water. Bring to a boil and boil gently for 2 minutes. Remove the pan from the heat, cover the pan, and set aside for 1 hour. Drain and cook as directed in the recipe.

And for those times when you have time only to open a can, just do that! Keep in mind that beans and legumes expand by about two-and-a-half times their size when cooked. Thus ½ cup dried black beans, for example, will be about 1½ cups when they are cooked and drained. So when replacing the dried beans in a recipe with canned, make sure you use two-and-a-half times the amount of dried beans called for. Note that a 15-ounce can holds about 1½ cups drained beans. Rinse and drain the canned beans thoroughly and simply add them to the dish whenever the *cooked* beans are added.

White Bean Lettuce Wraps

Makes 8 wraps; about 3 cups filling

I make lettuce wraps whenever I want a fresh, quick meal without a lot of bread. Plus, the cool crunch adds a dimension that makes it more fun to eat than a regular bread sandwich. You can form these ahead of time, but they are also really fun to serve so that people can form their own wraps. Place the bowl of white bean salad alongside a platter of crisp, fresh lettuce leaves, and you and your guests can compose and eat them on the spot. —DS

8 large romaine or Bibb lettuce leaves

1 (15-ounce) can cannellini or other white beans, rinsed and drained

1 small red onion, finely diced

1 large tomato, cored and diced

½ cup chopped fresh basil

2 tablespoons fresh lemon juice (from 1 lemon)

Sea salt and freshly ground black pepper

1. Trim and discard the bottom inch of the lettuce leaves. Set the leaves aside.

2. In a medium bowl, combine the beans, onion, tomato, basil, lemon juice, and salt and pepper to taste. Stir to mix well.

3. To form the wraps all at once place a lettuce leaf on your work surface and spoon some of the white bean mixture down the center rib. Roll up the leaf and place it seam-side down on a plate or platter. Or, if your leaves aren't wide enough to accommodate being rolled, simply roll up either side of the leaf and secure it with a toothpick across the filling.

4. Repeat with the remaining leaves and filling. Serve immediately.

RECIPES

Shiitake Mushroom Lettuce Wraps

Makes 8 wraps; about 2½ cups filling

I used to make this filling as a stir-fry and serve it over brown rice. That's always a great option, but at some point I realized that I really like the fresh flavor of the lettuce leaves wrapped around the earthy mushroom filling. As with the White Bean Lettuce Wraps on page 161, I often simply put out a platter of crisp lettuce and the filling and let my guests fill them and just fold them in half to eat right away. —DS

8 large romaine or Bibb lettuce leaves

8 ounces shiitake mushrooms, stemmed and sliced

2 cups finely chopped green cabbage

1 carrot, grated

2 green onions, white and light green parts thinly sliced

2 cloves garlic, minced

1 teaspoon grated peeled fresh ginger

2 teaspoons low-sodium soy sauce or tamari, plus more as needed

Freshly ground black pepper

1. Trim and discard the bottom inch from the lettuce leaves. Set the leaves aside.

2. Heat a large skillet over medium-high heat. Add the mushrooms, cabbage, and carrot, and cook, stirring occasionally and adding water 1 to 2 tablespoons at a time as needed to keep the vegetables from sticking, until crisp-tender, 2 to 3 minutes. Add the green onions, garlic, ginger, soy sauce, and pepper to taste, and cook for 1 minute, until heated through. Taste and add more soy sauce and pepper as desired.

3. To form the wraps all at once, place a lettuce leaf on your work surface and spoon some of the mushroom mixture down the center rib. Roll up the leaf and place it seam-side down on a plate or platter. Or, if your leaves aren't wide enough to accommodate being rolled, simply roll up either side of the leaf and secure it with a toothpick across the filling.

4. Repeat with the remaining leaves and filling. Serve immediately.

South-of-the-Border Pizza

Makes one (12-inch) pizza

I love pizza! And I like to surprise my guests by making pizzas you'll never find at your local pizza place. This one is always a hit with my friends—and me! —DS

1 (12-inch) precooked whole-grain pizza crust

1 cup Enchilada Sauce (page 271, or use store-bought)

1 cup cooked or canned black beans, rinsed and drained

1 red bell pepper, seeded and finely diced

1 large avocado, pitted, peeled, and diced

½ cup chopped fresh cilantro

1. Preheat the oven to 350°F.

2. Place the pizza crust on a pizza stone or large baking sheet. Spread the enchilada sauce over the crust. Sprinkle the black beans and bell pepper over the sauce.

3. Bake until the crust is lightly browned around the edges, about 15 minutes. Remove the pizza from the oven. Scatter the avocado over the pizza and sprinkle with the cilantro. Slice and serve.

RECIPES

Pizza with Creamed Spinach, Sun-Dried Tomatoes, Red Onion, and Olives

Makes two (12-inch) pizzas

I like a pizza that kicks with flavor, and this one does it for me. The creamy sauce is rich without the added fat that is in most cream sauces, and the sun-dried tomatoes and olives add a perfect tangy-salty punch. —DS

½ cup sun-dried tomatoes (not packed in oil)

1 (12-ounce) package firm or extra-firm silken tofu

1 (10-ounce) package frozen spinach, thawed

1 medium yellow onion, diced small

2 cloves garlic, minced

1 tablespoon dried dill

2 tablespoons nutritional yeast

Sea salt and freshly ground black pepper

2 (12-inch) precooked whole-grain pizza crusts

½ medium red onion, finely diced

1 cup pitted kalamata olives, halved

1. Place the sun-dried tomatoes in a small bowl and add enough warm water to cover. Set aside to soak until tender, about 30 minutes. Drain well. Finely chop the tomatoes and set aside.

2. Meanwhile, in a blender, puree the silken tofu until smooth. Set aside.

3. Preheat the oven to 350°F.

4. Lay a clean kitchen towel or several layers of paper towel on the counter and place the thawed spinach at the bottom of one short end. Roll up the spinach in the towel and, holding it over the sink, twist either end of the roll to squeeze out as much liquid from the spinach as you can. Unroll and set aside.

5. Heat a skillet over medium heat. Add the yellow onion and cook, stirring occasionally and adding water 1 to 2 tablespoons at a time as needed to keep the onion from sticking, until softened, about 5 minutes. Add the garlic and dill and cook until fragrant, about 1 minute. Stir

in the pureed tofu and the spinach along with the nutritional yeast. Cook to warm through, about 2 minutes. Season to taste with salt and pepper and remove from the heat.

6. Place the pizza crusts on pizza stones or large baking sheets. Divide the spinach mixture evenly between the crusts and spread it to cover the crusts evenly. Top with the chopped sun-dried tomatoes, red onion, and olives.

7. Bake until the edges are browned slightly and the pizzas are warmed all the way through, about 15 minutes. Slice and serve.

RECIPES

RECIPES

Tuscan White Bean Burgers

Makes 4 burgers

*Bursting with flavor, these are great on a bun with all the fixings—and
will never feel heavy. But if you'd like to keep the calorie density of the
meal even lower, serve the burgers on a bed of mixed greens. —DS*

1 cup sun-dried tomato halves
(not packed in oil)

½ cup cornmeal

2 cups cooked or canned
cannellini beans, rinsed and
drained

1 cup fresh basil, finely
chopped

½ medium red onion, minced

3 cloves garlic, minced

3 tablespoons arrowroot
powder

Sea salt and freshly ground
black pepper

4 whole-grain sandwich buns,
for serving

Ketchup, for serving

Lettuce, tomato, and red
onion slices, for serving

1. Place the sun-dried tomatoes in a small bowl
   and add enough warm water to cover. Set aside
   to soak until tender, about 30 minutes. Drain
   well. Finely chop the tomatoes and set aside.

2. Place the cornmeal in a bowl. Set aside. Have
   a nonstick baking sheet ready or line a regular
   baking sheet with parchment paper.

3. Place the beans in a large bowl and use a potato
   masher or fork to coarsely mash them, leaving
   some beans whole for texture. Add the chopped
   sun-dried tomatoes, basil, minced onion, garlic,
   arrowroot powder, and salt and pepper to taste.
   Stir until well mixed.

4. Divide the bean mixture into four equal
   portions. Shape each portion into a patty
   about 4 inches wide. Dredge each patty in
   the cornmeal and place on the baking sheet.
   Refrigerate for at least 1 hour.

5. Preheat the oven to 350°F.

6. Remove the burgers from the refrigerator and bake for 20 minutes. Use a spatula to carefully flip them, then continue to bake until firm and lightly browned, about 15 minutes more.

7. Serve on whole-grain buns topped with ketchup, lettuce, tomato, and red onion slices.

RECIPES

Navy Bean Hummus and Mixed Vegetable Pita Pockets

Makes 8 pita pockets; about 3 cups each hummus and mixed vegetables

Creamy, garlicky navy bean hummus and crunchy fresh vegetables are tucked into earthy, hearty whole wheat pitas in a perfect marriage of textures, colors, and flavors. —DT

FOR THE NAVY BEAN HUMMUS

1 cup dried navy beans, soaked (see page 160)

3 tablespoons fresh lime juice (from 2 limes)

1 clove garlic

½ teaspoon freshly ground black pepper

Sea salt

¼ cup finely chopped fresh cilantro

FOR THE MIXED VEGETABLES

1 medium beet, peeled and finely grated

1 medium tomato, cored and finely chopped

4 green onions, white and light green parts finely chopped

¼ cup grated carrot

½ cup finely chopped fresh cilantro

½ jalapeño, seeded and finely chopped

1. To prepare the hummus, place the soaked navy beans in a medium saucepan. Add 2 cups water and cook over high heat for 3 to 5 minutes. Reduce the heat and simmer, partially covered, until the beans are very tender, about 25 minutes. Remove the pan from the heat and let cool. Do not drain.

2. Transfer the cooled beans and their cooking liquid to a blender or food processor and add the lime juice, garlic, pepper, and salt to taste. Puree until smooth and well combined. Transfer to a medium bowl and fold in the cilantro. Cover and refrigerate until ready to serve. The hummus can also be stored in an airtight container in the refrigerator for 3 to 4 days.

3. To prepare the mixed vegetables, in a large bowl, combine the beet, tomato, green onions, carrot, cilantro, jalapeño, lime juice, sesame seeds, and salt to taste. Toss gently to mix.

1 tablespoon fresh lime juice
2 tablespoons sesame seeds
Sea salt

TO ASSEMBLE
4 whole-grain pita breads
2 cups salad greens

4. To assemble the pita pockets, lightly heat the pitas in a toaster or on a dry skillet over medium heat for about 20 seconds per side, making sure they do not get crisp.

5. Cut the pitas in half. Open one pocket and spread one-eighth of the hummus on one side of the interior. Spoon in some of the mixed vegetables and top with ¼ cup of the salad greens. Repeat with the remaining pita halves, hummus, salad mix, and greens. Serve immediately.

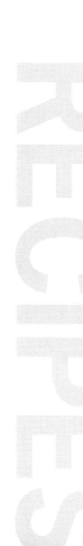

Spinach-Potato Tacos

Makes 4 tacos; about 6 cups filling

*Traditional Mexican tacos are much more than ground beef
and sour cream in a fried shell. There are many, many ways to
make tacos—in my opinion, this is one of the best. —DS*

2 large Yukon Gold potatoes,
  scrubbed and cut into small
  dice

1 (10-ounce) package frozen
  spinach, thawed

1 large onion, diced

1 medium poblano pepper,
  seeded and diced

2 cloves garlic, minced

2 teaspoons ground cumin

1 cup unsweetened,
  unflavored plant milk

3 tablespoons nutritional yeast

Sea salt and freshly ground
  black pepper

12 corn tortillas

½ cup chopped fresh cilantro

1. Place the potatoes in a medium saucepan and
   add water to cover. Bring to a boil, then reduce
   the heat to medium-low and simmer, covered,
   until the potatoes are tender when pierced with
   the tip of a sharp knife, 10 to 12 minutes. Drain
   well and set aside.

2. Meanwhile, lay a clean kitchen towel or several
   layers of paper towel on the counter and place
   the thawed spinach at the bottom of one short
   end. Roll up the spinach in the towel and,
   holding it over the sink, twist either end of the
   roll to squeeze out as much liquid from the
   spinach as you can. Unroll and set aside.

3. In a large skillet, cook the onion and poblano
   pepper over medium heat, stirring occasionally
   and adding water 1 to 2 tablespoons at a time
   as needed to keep the vegetables from sticking,
   until softened, 7 to 8 minutes. Add the garlic
   and cumin and cook until fragrant, about
   1 minute.

4. Add the reserved spinach and potatoes along with the plant milk and nutritional yeast. Season to taste with salt and pepper and cook until heated through, 2 to 3 minutes. Remove from the heat and set aside.

5. Meanwhile, heat a large nonstick skillet over medium heat. Add as many corn tortillas to the pan as will fit in a single layer and heat for a few minutes to warm the tortillas through. Remove them from the pan and set them aside, covered with a clean kitchen towel to keep warm. Repeat with the remaining tortillas.

6. To serve, place the tortillas on individual serving plates or a large platter and divide the potato mixture among them, spooning it onto the center of each. Sprinkle with cilantro and serve.

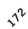

Asian Wraps

Makes 12 to 16 wraps

*Wraps like this one are great for packed lunches. It will stay fresh for
a few days if tightly wrapped and stored in the refrigerator. Use any
kind of mushroom you like—whether mild button, earthy shiitake,
or another that you prefer—all will be delicious here. —DT*

FOR THE NOODLES

7 ounces mung bean
vermicelli

4 ounces mushrooms, sliced
(about 1½ cups)

1 tablespoon finely chopped
peeled fresh ginger

1 cup finely chopped green
onions, white and light green
parts

3 tablespoons low-sodium
tamari

¼ teaspoon freshly ground
white or black pepper

FOR THE WRAPS

24 to 48 baby spinach leaves,
stems trimmed

10 large romaine lettuce
leaves

12 to 16 (8½-inch) rice paper
sheets

2 medium carrots, grated

1 large cucumber, peeled and
cut into thin strips about 3
inches long

1. Bring medium saucepan of water to a boil.
Add the vermicelli, cover the pan, and remove
the pan from the heat. Let stand until the
noodles are translucent, about 15 minutes.
(Alternatively, follow package instructions.)
Drain the noodles and use scissors to snip them
into shorter pieces (2 to 3 inches long). Set
aside (the noodles shouldn't sit too long or they
will stick together).

2. Meanwhile, in a large skillet with a lid,
combine the mushrooms, ginger, and ¼ cup
water and cook over medium heat, covered,
until the water is sizzling, about 2 minutes.
Add the green onions, tamari, and pepper and
cook, covered, until the mushrooms are tender
but still have bite, about 2 minutes. Add the
cooked vermicelli and mix gently, using a fork
to separate the noodles. Cook, uncovered, until
all the liquid has evaporated, about 2 minutes.
Transfer the mixture to a bowl and set aside to
cool.

1 cup finely chopped fresh
cilantro

1 cup finely chopped fresh
mint leaves

Wasabi Orange Sauce (page
264), for serving

3. Rinse the spinach leaves in cold water. Pat the leaves dry on a towel, or spin them dry in a salad spinner. The leaves need to be completely dry. Repeat with the lettuce leaves. Cut the center ribs out of the lettuce leaves and cut the remaining leaves into roughly 3 x 2-inch pieces.

4. Fill a medium bowl halfway with water and set it at your work area. Arrange the following items so they are also close at hand: the rice paper, a wooden cutting board, the noodle mixture, and the carrots, cucumber, cilantro, and mint.

5. To assemble the wraps, gently dip a sheet of rice paper in the bowl of water and let it soak for 20 seconds. Remove it from the water and place it on the cutting board. On the side closest to you, place 2 pieces of lettuce. Top with ⅓ to ½ cup of the noodle mixture. Place a few strips of carrot and cucumber on top. Sprinkle with cilantro and mint leaves. Cover the stuffing with 2 to 3 spinach leaves.

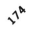

Asian Wraps *(cont.)*

6. Fold the edge of the rice paper that is closest to you over the stuffing and tuck it under on the other side, while pulling the package toward you. Hold the fold in place with one hand, and fold in the left and right sides of the paper with your other hand, to seal in the stuffing. Roll the wrap away from you until it is all rolled up. Set aside and repeat with the remaining rice paper and filling ingredients.

7. When all the wraps are assembled, you can serve them right away or transfer them to an airtight container and store in the refrigerator for 2 to 3 days. Let the wraps come to room temperature before serving.

8. When ready to serve, dip a sharp knife in water and use it to cut each wrap in half. Place the halves on a serving tray and serve the Wasabi Orange Sauce in a bowl alongside.

SIDE DISHES AND SALADS

Jamaican Fruited Rice Salad

Makes about 8 cups

This festive salad bursts with winning combinations of flavors, textures, and colors—sweet and savory; crunchy and juicy; bright orange, red, green, and yellow. That's probably why it's always a popular dish on a buffet table. —DS

4 cups cooked brown rice (see page 181), cooled

2 cups bite-size chunks fresh pineapple

1 (11-ounce) can mandarin orange slices packed in juice, drained

½ red bell pepper, seeded and finely diced

½ medium red onion, finely diced

1 small jalapeño, seeded and minced (optional)

½ small bunch cilantro, finely chopped

¼ cup fresh lime juice (from 2 to 3 limes)

¼ teaspoon ground allspice

Sea salt and freshly ground black pepper

1. In a large bowl, combine the rice, pineapple, mandarin slices, bell pepper, onion, jalapeño (if using), and cilantro. Toss lightly to combine.

2. In a separate small bowl, whisk together the lime juice, allspice, and salt and black pepper to taste. Pour the mixture over the rice mixture and toss until well coated. Cover and chill for 1 hour. Taste and adjust seasoning. Serve cold or at room temperature.

3. Store the salad in an airtight container in the refrigerator for up to 3 days.

RECIPES

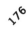

Beets and Barley Salad

Makes about 10 cups

The elements of this salad can be prepared ahead of time and assembled when you're ready to serve, which makes it a good option for a busy weekday evening or for serving guests. Go ahead and change the type of beets, greens, and seeds, depending on what's available, and create a completely new salad each time. Try yellow beets, baby kale or spinach, and sesame seeds, for instance, or red beets, arugula, and pumpkin seeds—there are so many delicious and beautiful variations! —DT

½ cup hulled barley

2 medium beets (about 10 ounces), scrubbed clean and quartered

2 tablespoons hulled sunflower seeds

6 cups chopped romaine lettuce

½ cup finely sliced green onions, white and light green parts

½ cup finely chopped fresh cilantro

2 tablespoons raisins

½ cup fresh orange juice (from 1 to 2 oranges)

1 tablespoon fresh lemon juice

⅛ teaspoon freshly ground black pepper

Sea salt

1. Place the barley in a medium bowl and cover generously with water. Set aside to soak for 3 hours.

2. Drain the barley and transfer it to a small saucepan. Add 2 cups water and bring to a boil over high heat. Boil for 5 to 7 minutes, then reduce the heat to maintain a simmer and cook, covered, until the barley is tender but not soft, about 25 minutes. It is important not to overcook the barley. Drain and set aside to cool to room temperature.

3. Meanwhile, place the beets in a medium saucepan and add cold water to cover. Bring to a boil over high heat, then reduce the heat to medium and simmer, partially covered, until the beets are tender when pierced with the tip of a sharp knife, about 30 minutes. Drain and

set aside just until cool enough to handle (the beets will be much easier to peel if they are warm). Peel the beets and cut them into bite-size pieces. Set aside.

4. Heat a small skillet over medium-high heat. Add the sunflower seeds and toast, shaking the pan occasionally, just until they smell toasty, 4 to 5 minutes. Immediately transfer them to a plate to cool.

5. In a large bowl, combine the barley and beets. Add the romaine, green onions, cilantro, raisins, orange juice, lemon juice, pepper, and salt to taste. Mix gently and taste for seasoning. Sprinkle the toasted sunflower seeds over the salad. Serve immediately.

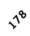

My Mama's Potato Salad

Makes about 14 cups

When I was a kid, I would only eat my mother's and my grandmother's potato salad—and I would certainly never eat potato salad from the grocery store. Try this recipe to find out why! —DS

8 medium red potatoes, scrubbed and chopped

1 (12-ounce) package firm or extra-firm silken tofu

2 tablespoons prepared yellow mustard

1 tablespoon Dijon mustard

4 cloves garlic, minced

1 tablespoon fresh lemon juice

½ teaspoon sea salt

¼ cup dill pickle relish

4 large stalks celery, finely diced

1 medium red onion, finely diced

Sea salt and freshly ground black pepper

1. Place the potatoes in a large pot and add cold water to cover. Bring the water to a boil over medium-high heat, then reduce the heat to medium-low and simmer the potatoes until just tender, 8 to 10 minutes. Drain the potatoes in a colander and rinse them under cold water until cool.

2. In a blender, combine the silken tofu, yellow mustard, Dijon mustard, garlic, lemon juice, and salt. Blend until smooth and creamy.

3. Transfer the mixture to a large bowl, add the relish, and stir well to combine. Add the celery, onion, and potatoes and toss gently to combine. Season with salt and pepper to taste.

4. Cover and chill for 1 hour. Taste and adjust seasoning before serving.

5. Store the salad in an airtight container in the refrigerator for up to 1 week.

No-Fuss Pasta Salad

Makes about 10 cups

There is no hard-and-fast rule for exactly which veggies or herbs to use in this recipe, although I do like this version very much. Go ahead and use your favorite no-oil dressing, your preferred frozen vegetables (or, you know, whatever is actually in your freezer tonight), and try other fresh herbs, such as tarragon or chives for a change. —DS

12 ounces whole-grain fusilli pasta

1 (16-ounce) bag mixed frozen vegetables

1 medium red onion, finely diced

Balsamic Vinaigrette (page 269) or 1 to 1½ cups store-bought oil-free Italian or balsamic dressing

1 cup chopped fresh basil

Sea salt and freshly ground black pepper

1. Bring a large pot of water to a boil and cook the pasta according to the package instructions. During the last 5 minutes of cooking, add the frozen vegetables to the pot with the pasta. Drain the pasta and vegetables and rinse under cold water until completely cool.

2. Transfer the mixture to a large bowl. Add the onion, dressing, and basil and toss to coat completely. Season with salt and pepper to taste. Serve chilled or at room temperature. Store the salad in an airtight container in the refrigerator for 2 to 3 days.

Mashed Potatoes and Gravy

Makes about 5 cups each potatoes and gravy

It's not hard to see why this dish represents comfort food for people of many different backgrounds. Its creamy, savory goodness is always a hit! —DT

¼ cup cashews

2 pounds russet potatoes (about 4 medium-large), scrubbed and chopped

2 cups cooked brown rice (see below)

8 ounces button mushrooms, sliced (about 4 cups)

4 cups low-sodium vegetable broth

½ teaspoon dried sage

½ teaspoon dried marjoram

½ teaspoon dried thyme

1 clove garlic, minced

2 tablespoons fresh lime juice (from 1 to 2 limes)

⅛ teaspoon freshly ground white or black pepper, plus ¼ teaspoon freshly ground black pepper

Sea salt

1. Place the cashews in a small bowl and cover with 1 cup water. Set aside to soak for 30 minutes.

2. Place the potatoes in a large saucepan and add cold water to cover. Bring to a boil over high heat, then reduce the heat to medium and cook until the potatoes are very tender when pierced with the tip of a sharp knife, about 20 minutes. Drain thoroughly and set aside to cool.

3. Meanwhile, in a saucepan, combine the rice, mushrooms, and vegetable broth. Bring to a boil over medium-high heat, then reduce the heat to medium and simmer until the mushrooms are tender, about 10 minutes. Remove from the heat and let cool slightly. Carefully transfer the mixture to a blender or food processor and blend until smooth. (Alternatively, leave the mixture in the pan and use an immersion blender to blend until smooth.)

4. If necessary, return the mixture to the pan. Add the sage, marjoram, thyme, garlic, lime juice, ⅛ teaspoon of the pepper, and salt to taste. Cook over medium heat for 10 minutes to blend

the flavors. Cover to keep the gravy warm and set aside.

5. Transfer the cashews and their soaking water to a clean blender. Add a pinch of salt and the remaining ¼ teaspoon pepper and blend until smooth. Pour the cashew cream over the potatoes and use a potato masher or handheld electric mixer to mash well. Taste and adjust the seasoning.

6. Serve the mashed potatoes topped with the gravy.

How to Cook Brown Rice

Place the rinsed rice (page 243) in a medium saucepan and add 2¼ times as much water as there is rice. Thus for 1 cup rice add 2¼ cups water.

Bring to a boil over high heat. Reduce the heat to low, cover the pan, and simmer for 45 minutes. Remove the pan from the heat and let stand, covered, for 5 to 10 minutes. Fluff with a fork before serving or using in another recipe.

The cooked yield will be roughly three times the amount of dry rice. Thus 1 cup uncooked rice will yield about 3 cups cooked.

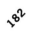
Millet Croquettes with Dill Dipping Sauce

Makes about 24 croquettes and about 1½ cups sauce

Millet is a unique grain that is prone to clumpiness and crunchiness if not cooked just so. Plus, it can be a little bland. You'd think that would make me run the other way, right? But those qualities are exactly what make it so perfect for this dish. Millet's sticky clumpiness is just what is needed to help the croquettes hold together; it forms a nice, crunchy crust when baked. And millet's neutral flavor is no issue at all, since there is plenty of that in all the vegetables in the croquettes and in the bright and tasty dipping sauce that is served alongside them. —DT

FOR THE DILL DIPPING SAUCE

½ cup dried navy beans, soaked (see page 160)

¼ cup cashews

½ cup fresh dill fronds

2 tablespoons fresh lemon juice (from 1 lemon)

2 cloves garlic

Pinch of freshly ground black pepper

Sea salt

FOR THE CROQUETTES

1½ cups millet

1 teaspoon ground turmeric

2 pounds white sweet potatoes (about 2 large), peeled and cut into 2-inch pieces

1 cup grated carrots

Be sure to grate the lemon zest for the croquettes before you juice the lemon for the dipping sauce. Look for sweet potatoes with white flesh; they are less sweet than the orange varieties, which makes them more suitable for this dish.

1. To make the dill dipping sauce, place the soaked navy beans in a small saucepan with 1 cup water. Bring to a boil over high heat, reduce the heat to medium, partially cover the pan, and simmer until very tender, about 20 minutes. Remove from the heat but do not drain. Set aside to cool to room temperature.

2. Meanwhile, place the cashews in a small bowl

1 cup minced green beans
(6 ounces)

½ cup minced green onions,
white and light green parts

2 tablespoons grated lemon
zest (from 3 to 4 lemons)

¼ teaspoon freshly ground
black pepper

Sea salt

and cover with ¾ cup water. Set aside to soak until softened, 1 to 2 hours.

3. In a blender, combine the cooked beans with their liquid and the cashews with their soaking water along with the dill, lemon juice, garlic, pepper and salt to taste. Blend until well combined, uniformly bright green, and creamy; this may take a few minutes. Taste and adjust the seasoning. Transfer the sauce to a covered container and chill until ready to serve. This sauce can be stored in the refrigerator for up to 5 days.

4. To make the croquettes, in a medium saucepan, bring 3 cups water to a boil over medium heat. Stir in the millet and turmeric and cook until the water returns to a boil. Cover the pan and simmer for 10 minutes (the liquid will probably not be completely absorbed yet). Remove from the heat and let stand, covered, for 10 minutes. Uncover and fluff the millet with a fork. Set aside to cool.

5. Meanwhile, place a steamer basket insert in a saucepan and fill the pan with a couple of inches of water (the water should not come above the level of the bottom of the steamer). Cover the pan and bring the water to a boil. Place the sweet potatoes in the steamer basket.

THE FORKS OVER KNIVES PLAN

RECIPES

Millet Croquettes with Dill Dipping Sauce *(cont.)*

Cover the pan and steam until the sweet potatoes are tender when pierced with a fork, 10 to 15 minutes. It is important not to overcook the potatoes. Transfer the potatoes to a large mixing bowl and mash them with a potato masher. Set aside to cool to room temperature.

6. When the mashed sweet potatoes and millet have cooled, add the millet to the bowl with the potatoes. Add the carrots, green beans, green onions, lemon zest, pepper, and salt to taste. Mix well but lightly. It is important to keep the mixture from getting dense and heavy.

7. Preheat the oven to 325°F. Line two baking sheets with parchment paper.

8. Using an ice cream scoop, place roughly ½-cup scoops of the millet mixture on the baking sheets, making sure they do not touch each other. You should have about 2 dozen croquettes.

9. Bake until the croquettes are lightly browned and crusty on the sides and bottom, about 30 minutes. Gently turn the croquettes over and continue to bake until nicely browned and crusty all around, about 30 minutes more; do not undercook or the croquettes will be crumbly. Serve hot, with the dipping sauce alongside.

Spicy French Fries

Makes 24 to 32 fries

Plain baked fries are certainly tasty enough, but once in a while it's nice to spice it up, as we do here. —DT

1 tablespoon onion powder

1½ teaspoons garlic powder

1½ teaspoons sweet paprika

1 teaspoon ground turmeric

1 teaspoon ground coriander

¼ teaspoon cayenne pepper

Sea salt

1½ pounds russet potatoes (3 or 4 medium-small), scrubbed

2 tablespoons fresh lemon juice (from 1 lemon)

Tomato ketchup and Dijon mustard, for serving (optional)

1. Preheat the oven to 350°F.

2. In a small bowl, stir together the onion powder, garlic powder, paprika, turmeric, coriander, cayenne, and salt to taste. Set aside.

3. Cut the potatoes into 1-inch-thick wedges. Pour ¼ cup water onto a rimmed baking sheet. Arrange the potato wedges on the tray, leaving plenty of room between them.

4. Bake for 20 minutes. Remove from the oven (leaving the oven on) and add ¼ cup water to the baking sheet to help loosen the potatoes; use a thin metal or wooden spatula to help release them. Sprinkle the mixed spices and the lemon juice over the potatoes, and mix gently but well to coat the potatoes evenly in the spices.

5. Return the pan to the oven and bake for 20 minutes. Add ¼ cup water to the pan and bake until the potatoes are tender when pierced with a fork, about 20 minutes more.

6. Serve the fries hot, with ketchup and Dijon mustard for dipping, if desired.

RECIPES

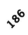
THE FORKS OVER KNIVES PLAN

Roasted Sweet Potato Wedges

Makes 8 wedges

The trick to achieving tender oil-free roasted sweet potatoes is to steam them before you put them in the oven. This precooking prevents the sweet potatoes from becoming overly chewy, which can happen when you roast them from raw without any oil. —DS

2 medium sweet potatoes (about 1½ pounds), peeled and quartered lengthwise

1 teaspoon granulated garlic

½ teaspoon ground cumin

½ teaspoon chili powder

½ teaspoon sea salt

½ teaspoon freshly ground black pepper

1. Preheat the oven to 425°F.

2. Place a steamer insert in a saucepan and add about 2 inches of water (the water should not come above the level of the bottom of the steamer). Cover the pan and bring the water to a boil. Place the potato wedges in the steamer, cover, and steam the potatoes until just tender, about 7 minutes.

3. Transfer the potato wedges to a nonstick baking sheet or a regular baking sheet lined with a silicone mat, arranging them in a single layer.

4. In a small bowl, combine the garlic, cumin, chili powder, salt, and pepper. Sprinkle the spice mixture evenly over the sweet potatoes.

5. Bake until brown and tender, 15 to 20 minutes, turning once during cooking. Serve hot.

Easy Baked Beans

Makes about 4 cups

When homemade barbecue sauce is in the refrigerator, this dish can be brought together in minutes. The barbecue sauce is what makes this dish; so if you don't have time to make it at home, make sure to use a great-tasting, low-sodium sauce in its place. Serve with roasted or grilled vegetables for a colorful and delicious meal. —DS

2 (15-ounce) cans pinto beans, rinsed and drained

2 cups Del's Basic Barbecue Sauce (page 270)

1. Preheat the oven to 325°F.
2. In a large bowl, combine the pinto beans and barbecue sauce and mix well. Transfer the beans to an 8 x 8-inch casserole dish.
3. Bake, uncovered, for 1 hour. Let stand for 5 minutes before serving.

Chickpeas in Greens

Makes about 4 cups

This is a great way to eat greens, especially bitter ones, in the winter. The dill and spinach are best kept as the dominant flavors, but otherwise, use whatever greens you like. The chickpeas need to be soaked for one to six hours, so be sure to plan ahead if you're using dried chickpeas. —DT

½ cup dried chickpeas, soaked (see page 160)

1 cup finely chopped leeks, white and light green parts

3 cloves garlic, minced

¼ bunch kale, stemmed, leaves finely chopped (about 1 cup)

½ bunch dandelion greens, stemmed, leaves finely chopped (about 1⅓ cups)

½ bunch spinach, stemmed, leaves finely chopped (about 3 cups)

½ bunch dill, tough stems removed, finely chopped (about ⅔ cup)

¼ bunch Swiss chard, stemmed, leaves finely chopped (about ¾ cup)

1 teaspoon finely chopped jalapeño

¼ teaspoon ground cloves

¼ teaspoon ground cinnamon

1 teaspoon fresh lemon juice

Sea salt

1. Place the soaked chickpeas in a small saucepan and add 1 cup water. Bring to a boil over high heat. Reduce the heat to medium and simmer, partially covered, until tender but not falling apart, 30 to 45 minutes. Drain and set aside.

2. Meanwhile, in a large saucepan or sauté pan, combine the leeks, garlic, and ½ cup water. Bring to a simmer over medium heat. Cover and cook for 10 minutes. Stir in the greens, jalapeño, cloves, cinnamon, lemon juice, salt to taste, and 1 cup water. Bring to a simmer, then cover the pan and cook, stirring occasionally, until the greens are very tender, about 10 minutes. Using an immersion blender, blend the greens until they are almost pureed. (Alternatively, transfer the greens to a standing blender and pulse until almost pureed.) Do not overblend; you don't want the greens to become a sauce.

3. If necessary, transfer the greens back to the pan. Stir in the chickpeas and cook over medium heat until heated through, 3 to 5 minutes. Taste and adjust the seasoning. Serve hot.

Hollywood Bowl Brown Rice Salad

Makes about 8 cups

This salad has been my favorite for a long time. It is filling yet refreshing, especially in the summer. There is no need for a separate dressing, and it can be made hours before serving, making it an ideal choice for a potluck or a picnic. Recently, I served this salad at a pre-show picnic at the Hollywood Bowl, and it was a big hit with my friends. —DT

1 cup brown rice

1 medium zucchini, finely chopped (about 1 cup)

1 medium-small cucumber, finely chopped (about 1 cup)

2 medium tomatoes, finely chopped (about 1 cup)

½ cup finely chopped green onions, white and light green parts

1 cup chopped fresh cilantro leaves

3 to 4 tablespoons fresh lemon juice (from about 2 lemons)

¼ teaspoon freshly ground black pepper

Sea salt

1. Rinse the rice and place it in a saucepan with 2 cups water. Bring the water to a boil over high heat. Reduce the heat to low, cover, and simmer until the rice is tender, about 45 minutes. Remove the pan from the heat and let stand, covered, for 10 to 15 minutes.

2. Transfer the rice to a large bowl and let it cool for a few minutes until no longer steaming. Add the zucchini, cucumber, tomatoes, green onions, cilantro, 3 tablespoons lemon juice, pepper, and salt to taste. Mix well. Taste and add more lemon juice or salt if desired. Cover and chill or let stand at room temperature for 30 minutes to allow the juices from the vegetables and the lemon juice to mix with the rice so that all the flavors meld. Taste and adjust seasoning.

3. Serve cold or at room temperature. Store the salad in an airtight container in the refrigerator for 2 to 3 days.

RECIPES

SOUPS AND STEWS

Mixed Bean and Vegetable Stew

Makes about 9 cups

This is a variation of a dish I discovered while traveling in Taos, New Mexico, where vegetable and bean stew was the only vegan item on the menu at a local restaurant. I loved the stew's unique earthy flavor, which I discovered came from a ground Peruvian chile called aji panca. *You can find it in markets that carry Peruvian products or it can be ordered online. Be careful—this chile is very hot. Alternatively, you can use ground smoked chipotle or cayenne pepper.* —DT

½ cup dried kidney beans, soaked (see page 160)

½ cup dried chickpeas, soaked (see page 160)

½ cup large-dice onion

1 cup large-dice tomatoes, plus 1 cup small-dice tomatoes

1 clove garlic

4 cups low-sodium vegetable broth

¾ cup diced scrubbed potato

1 cup ½-inch pieces trimmed green beans

1 cup small-dice carrot

1 cup sliced mushrooms

1 teaspoon ground cumin

1. Place the soaked kidney beans and chickpeas in a medium saucepan and add 3 cups water. Bring to a boil over high heat, then reduce the heat to medium-low and simmer, partially covered, until tender, 40 to 50 minutes. Remove from the heat and set aside; do not drain.

2. Meanwhile, in a blender or food processor, combine the onion, large-dice tomatoes, and garlic and blend into a paste. Transfer the paste to a large Dutch oven or soup pot. Stir in the vegetable broth. Bring to a boil over high heat and then adjust the heat as necessary to maintain a gentle boil for 5 minutes. Add the potato, cover the pan, and cook over medium

¼ teaspoon ground *aji panca,*
  ground smoked chipotle,
  or cayenne pepper

½ teaspoon apple cider
  vinegar

Sea salt

1 tablespoon finely chopped
  fresh cilantro, for serving

Cooked brown rice, for
  serving

heat for 10 minutes. Add water, if needed, to loosen the mixture to the consistency of a sauce.

3. Add the green beans, carrot, and mushrooms. Cover the pan and cook until the green beans are crisp-tender, 5 to 7 minutes. Add the reserved chickpeas and kidney beans with their cooking liquid along with the small-dice tomatoes, cumin, *aji panca,* vinegar, and salt to taste. Bring to a boil, then reduce the heat to medium and simmer for 15 minutes.

4. Remove from the heat and sprinkle the cilantro over the top. Serve hot, over brown rice.

RECIPES

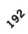

THE FORKS OVER KNIVES PLAN

30-Minute Chili

Makes about 7 cups

Every household I know has some version of chili in its recipe box. For my part, sometimes I make chili an all-day affair—cooking the beans from scratch, toasting the spices, and letting the chili simmer nice and slow for hours. And then there are the days I just need to get dinner on the table. This recipe is for those occasions, when delicious and fast are both *the order of the day. —DS*

1 large yellow onion, diced

1 large green bell pepper, seeded and diced

4 cloves garlic, minced

3 tablespoons mild chile powder

2 tablespoons ground cumin

1 tablespoon dried oregano

2 (15-ounce) cans pinto beans, rinsed and drained

1 (28-ounce) can diced tomatoes with their juice

2 cups vegetable broth

Sea salt and freshly ground black pepper

Cooked brown rice or whole-grain noodles for serving (optional)

1. In a Dutch oven or other deep saucepan, cook the onion and bell pepper over medium heat, stirring occasionally and adding water 1 to 2 tablespoons at a time as needed to keep the vegetables from sticking, until softened, about 5 minutes.

2. Add the garlic, chile powder, cumin, and oregano and cook for another minute. Add the beans, tomatoes, and broth. Bring to a simmer over medium-high heat. Reduce the heat, partially cover the pan, and simmer until the tomatoes start to break down and the mixture has thickened a little, about 20 minutes. Season with salt and pepper to taste.

3. Serve hot over rice or noodles, if desired.

RECIPES

Borscht (Beet Soup)

Makes about 6 cups

*Soup is the best way I know to prepare those larger beets that are
too dense to cook and eat as is. Even better is a soup like this one,
in which most of the ingredients are cooked together and then
blended and finished with some fresh herbs and a bit of citrus juice.
It's so easy and delicious, it feels a little like a cheat! —DT*

3 medium beets, peeled
and roughly chopped
(about 3 cups)

2 cups chopped scrubbed
potatoes

1 cup chopped onion

3 cloves garlic, chopped

¼ cup finely chopped fresh
parsley

1 tablespoon fresh lime juice
(from 1 lime)

⅛ teaspoon freshly ground
white pepper

Sea salt

1. In a large saucepan, combine the beets,
   potatoes, onion, garlic, and 2 cups water. Bring
   to a boil over high heat. Reduce the heat to
   medium-low and simmer, covered, until the
   vegetables are very tender, stirring occasionally,
   about 30 minutes. Let cool slightly.

2. Using an immersion blender, blend the soup
   until mostly smooth but with some chunky
   pieces for texture. (Alternatively, carefully
   transfer the soup to a standing blender and
   blend until mostly smooth.)

3. If necessary, pour the soup back into the
   saucepan. Add the parsley, lime juice, pepper,
   salt to taste, and 1 cup water. Bring to a simmer
   over medium heat and cook for 10 to 15 minutes
   to heat through and blend the flavors. Serve hot.

RECIPES

Lentil-Vegetable Stew

Makes about 7 cups

As this recipe is written, the vegetables will be cooked but crunchy. You can cook the lentils a bit longer if you prefer softer vegetables. I like this served as is, but for a heartier dish, serve it over steamed grains. —DT

1½ cups green or brown lentils, rinsed and soaked (see page 243)

1½ cups finely chopped leeks, white and light green parts

1 cup green beans, cut into ½-inch pieces before measuring

1 cup diced carrots

1 cup diced celery

1 tablespoon Italian seasoning

1 clove garlic, minced

½ teaspoon ground turmeric

Sea salt

1 tablespoon fresh lime juice (from 1 lime)

Steamed grains, for serving (optional)

1. Place the lentils in a large saucepan with the leeks and 3 cups water. Bring to a boil over high heat, then reduce the heat to medium and simmer until the lentils are just slightly tender, about 10 minutes.

2. Add the green beans, carrots, celery, Italian seasoning, garlic, turmeric, and salt. Partially cover the pan and cook over medium heat, stirring occasionally, until the vegetables are softened but still have good crunch, about 20 minutes. Add water as needed to keep the vegetables just covered.

3. Stir in the lime juice. Taste and adjust the seasoning. Serve hot, alone or spooned over grains, if desired.

Red Lentil Dal

Makes about 5 cups

This dal has a very traditional texture, where the lentils are mushy but still intact. For a soupier texture, blend the lentils in a blender before adding the lemon juice and cilantro. This is great served as is, or it can be the base for a variety of soups. Just add any vegetables, throw in some leftover cooked grains such as quinoa, brown rice, millet, or pasta, and you'll have a hearty one-meal dish. You can make a double batch and freeze it in smaller containers. Then whenever you have some leftover grains and a few wilting vegetables in your crisper drawer, defrost one of your frozen containers of dal and heat it up with your leftovers. Your meal will be ready in minutes! —DT

1½ cups red lentils, rinsed and soaked (see page 243)

1½ teaspoons grated peeled fresh ginger

1 teaspoon ground coriander

1 teaspoon onion powder

½ teaspoon ground turmeric

½ teaspoon ground cumin

½ teaspoon garlic powder

Sea salt

1 tablespoon fresh lemon juice (from 1 lemon)

1 tablespoon finely chopped fresh cilantro

Steamed rice or whole-grain bread, for serving

1. Place the lentils in a saucepan and add 4 cups water. Bring to a boil over high heat. Reduce the heat to medium and stir in the ginger. Cover the pan and simmer until the lentils are soft and have turned yellow, 15 to 20 minutes.

2. Add the coriander, onion powder, turmeric, cumin, garlic powder, salt to taste, and 1 cup water if the dal is very thick. Simmer for about 10 minutes more to blend the flavors.

3. Stir in the lemon juice and cilantro. Taste and adjust the seasoning. Serve hot, with rice or bread.

RECIPES

THE FORKS OVER KNIVES PLAN

RECIPES

Kale and Mung Bean Stew

Makes about 8 cups

This dish—with its blend of mung beans, fenugreek, and chipotle chiles—brings together a unique combination of Indian and Mexican flavors. Mung beans are a staple ingredient in Indian cooking, as well as in my pantry; I love how easy they are to cook and how quickly they can be transformed into a hearty stew (just be sure to plan ahead, as the dried beans must be soaked for one to six hours). Fenugreek seeds and greens are likewise used widely in Indian and Middle Eastern cuisines. In Indian cooking, fenugreek seeds are especially common in dishes with beans and lentils because they are believed to aid in digestion. Their distinct sweet and bitter flavor is often an integral aspect of Indian stews, curries, and dals. Chipotles are dried, smoked jalapeños; the meco variety has medium heat with a smoky, fruity, and spicy flavor that is especially welcome in this stew. —DT

½ cup finely chopped onion

1½ teaspoons grated peeled fresh ginger

2 cloves garlic, minced

2 teaspoons ground cumin

⅛ teaspoon whole or ground fenugreek seeds (optional)

1 brown meco chipotle chile

1½ cups dried mung beans, soaked (see page 160)

1 cup small-dice yellow bell pepper

2 cups finely chopped kale

2 tablespoons fresh lime juice (from 1 to 2 limes)

1. In a large soup pot or Dutch oven, combine the onion, ginger, garlic, cumin, fenugreek seeds (if using), chipotle, and 1 cup water. Bring to a simmer over medium heat and cook for 5 minutes.

2. Add the soaked mung beans, bell pepper, kale, lime juice, black pepper, salt to taste, and 4 cups water. Bring to a simmer, then cook, partially covered, until the mung beans are soft but not breaking down, 15 to 20 minutes.

3. Remove and discard the chipotle. Transfer 2 cups of the stew to a blender and puree; be

½ **teaspoon freshly ground**
  black pepper
Sea salt

careful that the hot soup does not overflow
the blender. (Alternatively, use an immersion
blender to blend the soup a bit in the pot. Don't
overblend. You want to leave some texture.)
Return the soup to the pot, if necessary, and
cook for 10 minutes more. Taste and adjust the
seasoning.

4. Serve hot.

RECIPES

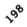
THE FORKS OVER KNIVES PLAN

Chickpea Flour Soup

Makes about 6 cups

Chickpea flour is a staple in my pantry because it is so versatile. It can be used to make batter for baked fritters (pakoras), savory pancakes, and cookies, and it's also good as a base for stews and as a thickener in soups. It has a hearty flavor and creamy texture that mixes well with the crunchiness of the vegetables in this soup. Chickpea flour is available in most health food stores and is stocked in the flour section; it is sometimes labeled as "gram flour." You will also find it in Southeast Asian and Persian stores. —DT

¼ cup sliced onion
½ teaspoon ground ginger
⅛ teaspoon celery seeds
⅛ teaspoon caraway seeds
⅛ teaspoon ground cumin
½ cup small-dice carrots
½ cup small-dice green beans
½ cup chickpea flour
1 cup small cauliflower florets
1 cup small broccoli florets
½ teaspoon garlic powder
Pinch of cayenne pepper
Pinch of freshly ground white or black pepper
Sea salt
1 teaspoon finely chopped fresh cilantro or chives
Baked potatoes or steamed brown rice, for serving (optional)

1. In a large soup pot, combine the onion, ginger, celery seeds, caraway seeds, cumin, and ½ cup water. Bring to a simmer and cook over medium-low heat for 5 minutes.

2. Add the carrots and green beans, cover the pot, and cook for 5 minutes more.

3. Meanwhile, in a medium bowl, whisk together the chickpea flour and 2 cups water until well blended and free of lumps. While stirring continuously, add the chickpea mixture to the soup, then add the cauliflower, broccoli, and 3 cups water.

4. Add the garlic powder, cayenne, pepper, and salt to taste. Bring to a simmer over medium heat, then reduce the heat to medium-low and cook, stirring often so as to avoid lumps, until

the chickpea flour no longer has a raw taste and the vegetables are tender, 10 to 15 minutes. The mixture will turn a richer yellow and thicken. Taste and adjust the seasoning.

5. Garnish with cilantro and serve hot as a soup, or with baked potatoes or brown rice.

Creamy Spinach Soup

Makes about 5 cups

This simple soup can be prepared pretty quickly. Its mild flavor and creamy texture make it a nice addition to any meal. —DT

¼ cup cashews

2 cups low-sodium vegetable broth

1 medium russet potato, scrubbed clean and cut into large dice

2 cups chopped leeks, white and light green parts

3 cloves garlic, chopped

¼ teaspoon dried thyme

3 or 4 bay leaves

1 bunch spinach, washed and stems trimmed

2 tablespoons fresh lemon juice (from 1 lemon)

¼ teaspoon freshly ground black pepper

Sea salt

1. Place the cashews in a small bowl and cover with 1 cup water. Set aside to soak for 30 minutes. Transfer the cashews and their soaking water to a blender and puree until smooth and creamy; this may take several minutes. Set aside.

2. In a soup pot, combine the broth, potato, leeks, garlic, thyme, and bay leaves and bring to a boil over high heat. Reduce the heat to medium, cover the pot, and simmer until the potato is very tender, about 15 minutes.

3. Add the spinach and 1 cup water. Cover and cook over medium heat until the spinach leaves have wilted, about 5 minutes. Let cool slightly.

4. Remove and discard the bay leaves. Carefully transfer the soup to a blender or food processor, working in batches if necessary (do not overfill the blender), and puree until smooth. (Alternatively, use an immersion blender to puree the soup in the pot until smooth.)

5. Pour the soup back into the pot. Whisk in the cashew cream, lemon juice, pepper, and salt to taste and bring to a boil. Taste and adjust the seasoning. Serve hot.

Cream of Broccoli Soup

Makes about 9 cups

This soup provides the enormous satisfaction of transforming a large amount of broccoli into a luscious and creamy soup. —DT

2 pounds broccoli with stems

½ medium onion, roughly chopped

1 small potato, scrubbed and roughly chopped

1 teaspoon garlic powder

2 cups fresh or frozen green peas

⅛ teaspoon freshly ground black pepper

3 tablespoons fresh lemon juice (from 1 to 2 lemons)

1 tablespoon finely chopped fresh dill

Sea salt

1. Cut the broccoli into large pieces, keeping the florets separate from the stems. Peel any very tough stems. Place the stems in a large soup pot and add the onion, potato, garlic powder, and 3 cups water. Bring to a boil over high heat. Reduce the heat to medium and cook for 10 minutes.

2. Add the broccoli florets and the peas to the pot and cook until the broccoli is very tender, about 15 minutes.

3. Carefully transfer the soup to a blender, working in batches if necessary, and blend until smooth. (Alternatively, use an immersion blender to puree the soup in the pot until smooth.)

4. Return the soup to the pot, if necessary. Add water if necessary, so that the consistency of the soup is moderately thick. Stir in the lemon juice, dill, and salt to taste and bring to a boil.

5. Serve hot.

RECIPES

Butternut Squash Soup with Sautéed Green Peas and Pesto Sauce

Makes about 7 cups

This soup is so good, even if you only have enough time to make just one of the two beautiful and tasty toppings. However, I highly recommend that you go ahead and make both whenever you can, so that you can fully enjoy the flavor and textural contrast between the mildly sweet, silky smooth soup; the tangy green onion topping; and the grassy, nutty, bright taste of the fresh pesto. The combination transforms three simple parts into a deliciously complex whole. —DT

FOR THE SOUP

10 cups cubed, peeled, and seeded butternut squash (3 pounds)

FOR THE TOPPING

2 cups fresh or frozen green peas

1½ cups finely chopped green onions, white and light green parts

2 tablespoons fresh lime juice (from 1 to 2 limes)

Pinch of freshly ground black pepper

Sea salt

FOR THE PESTO SAUCE

2 cups packed fresh basil leaves

¼ cup pine nuts

1. To make the soup, place the squash in a large sauté pan with a lid and add 2 cups water. Bring to a boil over high heat. Reduce the heat to medium, cover the pan, and simmer until the squash is soft, about 20 minutes. Remove from the heat and let cool; do not drain. Transfer the squash and its cooking water to a blender or food processor and blend until smooth. Set aside.

2. Meanwhile, to make the topping, bring a small saucepan of water to a boil. Add the peas and boil until very tender, 5 to 7 minutes. Drain the peas and let cool.

3. In a sauté pan, cook the green onions over medium heat in 2 to 3 tablespoons of water, until they are tender and the water has

1 clove garlic
¼ teaspoon freshly ground
black pepper
Sea salt

evaporated, about 5 minutes. Add the peas, lime juice, pepper, and salt to taste. Cook until the ingredients are blended and warmed through, about 2 minutes. Taste and adjust the seasoning. Set aside.

4. To make the pesto sauce, place the basil, pine nuts, garlic, pepper, and salt in a blender or food processor and blend until smooth. Transfer to a small dish and stir in 1 or 2 tablespoons of water to make a creamy paste.

5. When ready to serve, warm the soup until hot and ladle it into bowls. Top each serving with a spoonful of sautéed green pea topping and place a spoonful of the pesto sauce on top. Serve hot.

THE FORKS OVER KNIVES PLAN

RECIPES

Potato-Vegetable Chowder

Makes about 11 cups

Nothing warms the bones on a cold day like a big bowl of piping-hot soup. Try using root vegetable like parsnips or turnips for a nice change of pace. —DS

1 medium yellow onion, finely chopped

2 stalks celery, finely chopped

2 medium carrots, finely chopped

2 teaspoons dried thyme

1 bay leaf

2 large red potatoes, scrubbed and cubed

3½ cups vegetable broth

1 (16-ounce) bag frozen mixed vegetables

3 tablespoons arrowroot powder

2½ cups unsweetened, unflavored plant milk

Sea salt and freshly ground black pepper

1. In a large saucepan, cook the onion, celery, and carrots over medium heat, stirring occasionally and adding water 1 to 2 tablespoons at a time as needed to keep the vegetables from sticking, until beginning to brown, 7 to 8 minutes. Add the thyme and bay leaf and cook for 1 minute.

2. Add the potatoes and vegetable broth. Bring to a simmer. Partially cover the pot and simmer until the potatoes are just tender, about 10 minutes.

3. Add the frozen vegetables and return to a simmer. Partially cover the pot and simmer until the vegetables are tender, about 10 minutes.

4. Meanwhile, in a medium bowl, combine the arrowroot powder and plant milk and whisk until well blended. Add the mixture to the pot with the vegetables and stir until well combined. Simmer gently until the soup has thickened.

5. Season to taste with salt and pepper and cook for 5 minutes more. Remove and discard the bay leaf.

6. Serve hot.

Lima Bean Soup

Makes about 10 cups

The founder of Forks Over Knives, Brian Wendel, had his first taste of lima bean soup while he was traveling along the coast of California. He loved the creamy texture and mild taste of the lima beans in a soup also chock-full of hearty vegetables. Now that I've come up with our own Forks Over Knives rendition, I must say that I share his enthusiasm for the combination. The soup comes together easily whether you use canned or frozen limas. It's great to make for a weeknight dinner, but it tastes even better the day after you make it. —DS

1 large yellow onion, diced

2 large carrots, diced

2 large stalks celery, diced

¼ cup tomato paste

3 cloves garlic, minced

2 teaspoons dried thyme

1 teaspoon dried sage, crumbled

2 large turnips, peeled and cubed

4 cups rinsed and drained canned lima beans, or use frozen

6 cups vegetable broth

Sea salt and freshly ground black pepper

1. In a large soup pot or Dutch oven, cook the onion, carrots, and celery over medium heat, stirring occasionally and adding water 1 to 2 tablespoons at a time as needed to keep the vegetables from sticking, until the onions are translucent and starting to brown, 8 to 10 minutes. Add the tomato paste, garlic, thyme, and sage and cook for 1 minute.

2. Add the turnips, lima beans, and vegetable broth and bring to a boil over high heat. Reduce the heat to medium and simmer the soup until thickened, about 15 minutes. Season to taste with salt and pepper and cook until the vegetables are completely cooked, about 10 minutes.

3. Serve hot.

Tortilla Soup

Makes about 8 cups

Many traditional Mexican dishes are easy to adapt to a fully plant-based diet. This tortilla soup is a great example. Whenever I cook it, the whole house fills with a delightful aroma, a hint of the robust and delicious flavor that is on the way. —DT

6 corn tortillas

6 large tomatoes, halved

2 red bell peppers, halved

8 ounces mushrooms, roughly chopped (about 2 cups)

½ yellow onion, roughly chopped

3 cloves garlic, roughly chopped

2 teaspoons ground cumin

2 dried chipotle chiles

5 to 7 sprigs fresh cilantro

2 teaspoons smoked mild paprika

½ teaspoon chili powder

Sea salt

2 cups fresh or frozen corn

2 cups fresh or frozen green peas

½ cup thinly sliced green onions, white and light green parts, for serving

½ cup chopped fresh cilantro, for serving

1 avocado, diced, for serving

1. Preheat the oven to 400°F. Line a baking sheet with parchment paper.

2. Cut the corn tortillas into ¼-inch-wide strips and spread the strips on the baking sheet. Bake until crispy, 20 to 25 minutes. Set aside.

3. Meanwhile, in a large soup pot or Dutch oven place the tomatoes, bell peppers, mushrooms, onion, garlic, cumin powder, chipotle chiles, cilantro sprigs, and 1 cup water. Bring to a boil over high heat. Reduce the heat to medium, cover the pan, and simmer, stirring occasionally, until the vegetables are tender, 20 to 30 minutes.

4. Remove and discard the chiles and cilantro sprigs. Transfer the soup to a blender or food processor. Blend until smooth. Pour the mixture back into the pan. Add the smoked paprika, chili powder, salt to taste, and 2 cups water. Bring to a boil over medium-high heat, then reduce the heat to medium and simmer until the soup thickens, about 10 minutes.

RECIPES

½ cup chopped tomatoes,
for serving (optional)

½ Meyer or other lemon, for
serving

5. Add the corn and green peas and cook until tender but still crisp, about 5 minutes.

6. To serve, garnish each serving of soup with green onions, cilantro, avocado, tomatoes, if using, and the reserved corn strips. Squeeze some lemon juice on top.

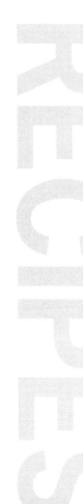

White Bean Stew with Herbed Pancakes

Makes about 6 cups stew and 8 pancakes

To me, a hot, opened-face sandwich is always a welcome meal, but especially on a cool evening. The "bread" for this particular sandwich is actually a savory pancake that is especially welcoming and fresh, because it goes straight from the skillet to the plate. —DT

FOR THE STEW

1 cup dried navy beans, soaked (see page 160)

1 packed cup chopped leeks (white and light green parts)

1 big clove garlic, minced

1 cup diced carrots

1 cup diced green beans

1 cup cauliflower florets

1 cup diced tomatoes

1 cup diced red bell pepper

2 tablespoons Italian seasoning

1 teaspoon chili

2 tablespoons white wine vinegar

Sea salt

FOR THE PANCAKES

¾ cup sorghum flour

¾ cup oat flour

2 tablespoons cashew or almond flour

1 teaspoon ground chia or flaxseeds

1. To prepare the stew, place the soaked beans in a large saucepan. Add the leeks, garlic, and 3 cups water. Bring to a boil, then reduce the heat to medium and simmer, partially covered, until the beans are just tender, 15 to 20 minutes. Add the carrots, green beans, cauliflower, tomatoes, bell pepper, and Italian seasoning. Cook until the beans and vegetables are completely cooked, 15 to 20 minutes. Add the vinegar and salt to taste. Cook for 2 to 3 minutes.

2. Meanwhile, prepare the pancakes. In a large mixing bowl, whisk together the sorghum flour, oat flour, cashew flour, chia seeds, garlic powder, marjoram, oregano, thyme, baking soda, baking powder, and a generous pinch of salt. Pour in the vinegar and 1½ cups water and stir gently until well blended.

3. Heat a griddle or large nonstick pan over medium heat until a few droplets of water dropped in the pan jump and sizzle.

½ teaspoon garlic powder

½ teaspoon dried marjoram

½ teaspoon dried oregano

½ teaspoon dried thyme

¼ teaspoon baking soda

1 teaspoon baking powder

Sea salt

1½ teaspoons apple cider vinegar

4. Spoon ¼ cup for each pancake onto the pan. Cook until the edges look dry and the bottoms are crisp and lightly browned, 5 to 7 minutes. Using a spatula, turn the pancakes over and cook for 5 minutes more. Repeat with the remaining batter. (If the batter becomes too thick as it sits, stir in 1 to 2 tablespoons water to return it to a pourable consistency.)

5. For each serving, ladle some hot stew over the pancakes and serve hot.

RECIPES

RECIPES

Chickpea Chili on Baked Potatoes

Makes about 6 cups chili and 4 potatoes

At a deli one afternoon I ordered a tomato-vegetable soup and a baked potato. When I received the two items, they looked like they belonged together, so I poured the soup right over the potato. The result? A tasty new meal and the spark that led to all sorts of new dishes that turn baked potatoes into the base for soups, stews, and chilis. This is one of my favorites. —DT

1 cup dried chickpeas, soaked (see page 160)

4 large russet potatoes (about 2 pounds), scrubbed

4 cups diced tomatoes

2 cups diced red bell pepper

8 ounces button mushrooms, trimmed and diced (about 2 cups)

1 cup finely chopped red onion

2 cloves garlic, minced

1 teaspoon ground cumin

2 teaspoons dried oregano

1½ cups diced celery

1 cup finely chopped green bell pepper

1 cup fresh or frozen corn

2 tablespoons white wine vinegar

1 tablespoon fresh lemon juice

1 teaspoon smoked paprika

¼ teaspoon chili powder or to taste

¼ cup finely chopped fresh cilantro, for serving

Sea salt

1. Place the soaked chickpeas in a medium saucepan and add 3 cups water. Bring to a boil over high heat. Reduce the heat to medium and simmer, partially covered, until they are tender to the bite but not falling apart, 30 to 45 minutes. Add water as necessary to keep the chickpeas covered. Drain and set aside.

2. Preheat the oven to 450°F.

3. Use a fork to poke holes in the potatoes in several places. Place them on a baking sheet and bake until a fork goes through to the center easily, 40 to 60 minutes. (If the potatoes are baked before the stew is ready, turn the oven off and let the potatoes stand in hot oven until ready to serve.)

4. Meanwhile, in a large saucepan, place the tomatoes, red bell pepper, mushrooms, onion, garlic, cumin, and oregano. Cook over medium heat for 20 minutes, stirring occasionally. (The juices from the onion and tomatoes will be enough to keep the sauce from burning.)

RECIPES

Transfer the sauce to a blender or food processor and blend until smooth. Set aside.

5. To the same saucepan, add 3 cups water. Add the reserved cooked chickpeas, the celery, green bell pepper, and corn. Bring to a boil over high heat. Add the reserved tomato sauce, vinegar, lemon juice, paprika, chili powder, half of the cilantro, and salt to taste. Cook until the vegetables are tender and the chili thickens, 15 to 20 minutes.

6. Use a sharp knife to cut down the length of each potato and spread them open. Pour a good helping of the chili over each potato. Garnish with cilantro and serve hot.

Pasta e Fagioli

Makes about 8 cups

I like to use rice pasta and white beans for this dish, as I have here, but feel free to substitute or add any cooked pasta, grain, or beans—as well as swapping out the carrots and green beans for whatever vegetable is in season right now—to create something uniquely your own. —DT

¾ **cup rice macaroni pasta**

2 **cups low-sodium vegetable broth**

1 **(15-ounce) can diced tomatoes with their juice**

½ **cup finely chopped onion**

1 **(15-ounce) can low-sodium white beans, rinsed and drained**

1 **cup small-dice carrots**

1 **cup diced green beans**

1 **teaspoon dried oregano**

1 **teaspoon dried basil**

1 **teaspoon white wine vinegar**

⅛ **teaspoon red pepper flakes**

1. Bring a medium saucepan of water to a boil. Add the macaroni and cook according to the package instructions until al dente (avoid overcooking). Drain well and set aside.

2. Meanwhile, in another saucepan, combine the vegetable broth, diced tomatoes, and onion. Bring to a simmer over medium heat, then cover the pan and cook for 10 minutes.

3. Add the white beans, carrots, green beans, oregano, basil, and 2 cups water. Bring to a simmer over medium-high heat, then cover and cook until the green beans and carrots are completely cooked, about 20 minutes.

4. Stir in the cooked pasta along with the vinegar and red pepper flakes. Stir well and cook for 5 minutes to heat through and blend the flavors. Taste and adjust the seasonings. Serve hot.

CASSEROLES

Sweet Potato Lasagna

Makes one (9 × 13-inch) lasagna

For this dish use white-fleshed sweet potatoes, which can have brown, purple, or reddish-orange skin (they may be labeled as yams, as sweet potatoes often are). Their flesh is starchier and drier than the moister, sweeter orange-colored varieties, such as the "garnet" or "jewel" type; and they are better in this dish because they will hold their texture without becoming overly moist or runny. You can find these sweet potatoes in most well-stocked grocery store produce departments and at farmers' markets. —DT

This dish is ideal to serve to a group. It has all sorts of different tastes and textures.
Serve it with a salad for a complete meal.

FOR THE CASHEW CHEESE

1 cup cashews

1½ tablespoons nutritional yeast

2 tablespoons fresh lime juice (from 1 to 2 limes)

¼ teaspoon garlic powder

¼ teaspoon sea salt

¼ teaspoon freshly ground black pepper

1. To prepare the cashew cheese, place the cashews in a small bowl and add at least 1 cup water. Set aside to soak until softened, 1 to 2 hours. Drain the cashews and place them in a blender with the nutritional yeast, lime juice, garlic powder, salt, pepper, and ¾ cup water. Blend until the mixture is smooth and has the consistency of cream cheese. Transfer the cashew cheese to a zip-top bag or a squeeze bottle and set aside.

Sweet Potato Lasagna *(cont.)*

FOR THE SWEET POTATO FILLING

3 pounds white-fleshed sweet potatoes (4 to 5 medium), peeled and cut into big pieces

1 tablespoon fresh lime juice (from 1 lime)

Sea salt

FOR THE SAUTÉED GREENS

2 cups finely chopped leeks, white and light green parts

12 ounces button mushrooms, finely chopped (4 cups)

2 small cloves garlic, minced

Sea salt

1 bunch Swiss chard, stemmed and finely chopped (about 4 cups)

1 bunch spinach, stemmed and finely chopped (about 4 cups)

FOR THE TOMATO SAUCE

3 medium tomatoes, diced (about 3 cups)

1 cup diced red onion

2 (6-ounce) cans tomato paste

2 pitted dates

2 cloves garlic

1 tablespoon dried oregano

1 tablespoon dried basil

⅛ teaspoon freshly ground black pepper

Sea salt

1 pound rice lasagna pasta noodles (16 noodles)

2. Meanwhile, to prepare the sweet potato filling, place a steamer basket insert in a saucepan filled with about 2 inches of water. Bring the water to simmer and add the sweet potatoes. Cover the pan and steam until tender when pierced with the tip of a sharp knife, 15 to 17 minutes. Transfer the sweet potatoes to a large bowl.

3. Use a potato masher to mash the sweet potatoes. Add the lime juice and salt and mix well. Set aside.

4. To prepare the sautéed greens, in a sauté pan, combine the leeks and ¼ cup water. Cover and cook over low heat until the leeks are very soft, about 15 minutes. Add the mushrooms, garlic, and salt. Cook, covered, over medium heat until the mushrooms are soft, 5 to 7 minutes. Add the Swiss chard and the spinach and cook, uncovered, until the greens are tender, 5 to 7 minutes. Remove from the heat and let cool.

5. To prepare the tomato sauce, in a blender or food processor, combine the tomatoes, onion, tomato paste, dates, garlic, and 1 cup water. Blend until smooth. Transfer the mixture to a saucepan and add the oregano, basil, pepper, a generous pinch of salt, and 2 cups water. Cook over medium heat for 40 minutes. Taste for seasoning and set aside.

6. Bring a large pot of water to a boil. Cook the pasta according to the instructions on the package. Drain thoroughly. Lay out the noodles on a wire rack or towel, making sure they are spread out and not layered on top of one another. Let cool.

7. Preheat the oven to 350°F.

8. To assemble the lasagna, in the bottom of a 9 x 13-inch baking pan that is at least 2 inches deep, spread 1½ cups of the tomato sauce. Arrange a layer of 4 lasagna noodles on top, overlapping each noodle slightly with the one that was laid down before.

9. Top with half of the mashed sweet potatoes, then another layer of 4 noodles. Spread all of the sautéed greens on top. Pipe half of the cashew cheese on top (if the cashew cheese is in a zip-top bag, just snip off one corner so you can pipe the cheese over the greens).

10. Arrange a layer of 4 pasta noodles on top of the cheese. Spread half of the remaining tomato sauce over the pasta. Spread the remaining sweet potatoes on top.

11. Arrange the last layer of pasta atop the sweet potatoes. Spread the remaining tomato sauce on top. Pipe the remaining cheese over the sauce in a fun zigzag or swirling pattern.

12. Bake until the cheese on top is lightly browned and the sauce is bubbling along the sides of the pan, about 45 minutes. Let stand for 5 minutes before serving.

13. Serve hot.

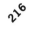
THE FORKS OVER KNIVES PLAN

Rice Casserole with Lentils and Sautéed Vegetables

Makes one (9 × 13-inch) casserole

This dish is a real crowd-pleaser, and is especially good for big gatherings like Super Bowl parties. I love it with rice, but it's also really good with pasta. Both options are given below. The lentils need to be soaked for at least six hours, so be sure to plan ahead. —DT

FOR THE CASHEW CRUMBLE CHEESE

½ cup cashews

3 tablespoons nutritional yeast

½ teaspoon low-sodium tamari or soy sauce, Bragg's liquid aminos, or fresh lime juice

1 cup brown lentils, rinsed and soaked (see page 243)

1 teaspoon Italian seasoning

Sea salt

1½ cups brown rice, or 3 cups penne pasta

FOR THE SAUTÉED VEGETABLES

2 medium sweet potatoes, scrubbed and cut into ½-inch dice

¼ medium cabbage, chopped into ½-inch pieces

½ medium red onion, cut into ½-inch dice

2 cloves garlic, minced

1. To make the cashew crumble cheese, in a food processor, grind the cashews into a meal (do not overprocess into cashew butter). Transfer them to a small bowl, and mix in the nutritional yeast. Little by little, add the liquid of your choice, stirring with a fork so that the mixture does not form clumps. The mixture should be crumbly. Set aside to dry until ready to use.

2. Place the soaked lentils in a medium saucepan with the Italian seasoning, salt, and 1 cup water. Bring to a boil over high heat, then reduce the heat to medium, and cook, covered, until the lentils are cooked but still firm, about 15 minutes. Be careful not to overcook them. Set aside.

3. Meanwhile, if using rice, place it in a medium saucepan with 2½ cups water. Bring to a boil and stir once. Cover the pan, reduce the heat

RECIPES

1 teaspoon dried basil

2 cups low-sodium vegetable broth

2 medium zucchini, cut into ½-inch dice

1 bell pepper, any color, seeded and cut into ½-inch dice

1 tablespoon arrowroot powder

FOR THE TOMATO SAUCE

½ cup finely chopped onion

1 (15-ounce) can diced tomatoes with their juice

1 teaspoon dried basil

⅛ teaspoon freshly ground white or black pepper

Sea salt

1 cup roughly chopped fresh basil

to low, and simmer, covered, until the rice is cooked, about 25 minutes. Remove from the heat and let stand, covered, for 5 minutes. Remove the cover and fluff the rice. Set aside.

4. If using pasta, bring a large saucepan of water to a boil. Add the pasta and cook according to the package instructions until the pasta is al dente. Drain thoroughly and set aside.

5. Preheat the oven to 350°F.

6. To prepare the sautéed vegetables, in a skillet with a lid, combine the sweet potatoes, cabbage, onion, garlic, dried basil, and 1½ cups of the vegetable broth. Cover and cook over medium heat, stirring occasionally, until the sweet potatoes are almost tender but still resist a bit when pierced with a knife, 15 to 20 minutes.

7. Add the zucchini and bell pepper and cook, uncovered, until the vegetables are completely softened, about 10 minutes.

8. In a small bowl, combine the remaining ½ cup vegetable broth and the arrowroot powder. Whisk until blended. Pour the mixture over the vegetables and stir gently to coat them. Cook over medium-low heat, uncovered, for

Rice Casserole with Lentils and Sautéed Vegetables *(cont.)*

5 minutes. Remove from the heat and set aside.

9. Meanwhile, prepare the tomato sauce. In a saucepan, combine the onion and ½ cup water. Cover and cook over high heat until the onions are very soft, about 10 minutes.

10. Add the tomatoes, dried basil, pepper, and salt, and cook over medium heat until the sauce thickens a bit and the flavors merge, about 15 minutes. Remove the pan from the heat and stir in the fresh basil. Taste and adjust the seasoning. Set aside.

11. Spread the rice or pasta in a 9 x 13-inch baking pan that is 2 inches deep. Layer the lentils over the rice to cover completely. Spread the sautéed vegetables over the lentils. Spoon the tomato sauce over the vegetables. Spread the cashew crumble cheese all over the top.

12. Bake until the cashew cheese turns light brown, about 20 minutes.

13. Serve hot.

Tex-Mex Bean and Cornbread Casserole

Makes one (9 × 13-inch) casserole

My dad made a version of this dish when I was a kid that had bacon and sausage, and the cornbread was always from a box mix. Naturally, we loved it! Today, I far prefer my interpretation of this family favorite, which is full of all the good taste and none of the bad ingredients. Note that you'll need to make a double batch of the barbecue sauce for this recipe. —DS

1 large yellow onion, diced

1 large green bell pepper, seeded and diced

1 (15-ounce) can pinto beans, rinsed and drained

1 (15-ounce) can black beans, rinsed and drained

1 (15-ounce) can chickpeas, rinsed and drained

5 cups Del's Basic Barbecue Sauce (page 270) or use store-bought

1 cup whole wheat pastry flour

1 cup cornmeal

1 tablespoon baking powder

½ teaspoon sea salt

1½ cups unsweetened, unflavored plant milk

½ cup unsweetened applesauce

¼ cup maple syrup (optional)

1. Preheat the oven to 350°F.

2. Heat a large sauté pan over medium heat. Add the onion and bell pepper and cook, stirring occasionally and adding water 1 to 2 tablespoons at a time as needed to keep the vegetables from sticking, until softened, about 5 minutes. Add the pinto beans, black beans, chickpeas, and barbecue sauce and simmer over medium-low heat for 15 minutes, stirring occasionally. Pour the bean mixture into a 9 x 13-inch baking dish and set aside.

3. In a medium bowl, combine the flour, cornmeal, baking powder, and salt. Whisk to combine. Make a well in the center of the dry ingredients and add the plant milk, applesauce, and maple syrup (if using). Whisk the wet ingredients together and gently fold in the flour mixture just to combine. Do not overmix.

4. Spoon the batter over the beans in the baking dish and carefully spread it so that it evenly covers the surface. Bake until the cornbread is firm to the touch and slightly browned, 20 to 25 minutes. Let stand for 5 minutes before serving hot.

RECIPES

Potato Enchiladas

Makes one (9 × 13-inch) pan

*Enchiladas stuffed with a flavorful potato-and-mushroom filling
and covered in spicy sauce and creamy cashew cheese is nothing
less than the most heavenly kind of comfort food. —DT*

FOR THE FILLING

2 pounds Yukon Gold
potatoes, scrubbed and
halved

1 cup low-sodium vegetable
broth

6 ounces mushrooms, finely
chopped (about 2 cups)

1 teaspoon dried oregano

1 teaspoon ground cumin

Sea salt

¾ cup frozen corn

¾ cup frozen green peas

Enchilada Sauce (page 271),
warmed

12 (7- to 8-inch) or 18 (6-inch)
wheat or corn tortillas

Half recipe Cashew Cheese
(page 213)

1. To prepare the filling, place the potatoes in a
   large saucepan and cover with cold water. Bring
   to a boil over high heat, then reduce the heat to
   medium and cook, partially covered, until the
   potatoes are tender when pierced with the tip
   of a sharp knife, about 30 minutes. Drain well
   and transfer the potatoes to a large bowl. Mash
   the potatoes coarsely. Set aside.

2. In a skillet, heat the vegetable broth. Add
   the mushrooms, oregano, cumin, and salt to
   taste. Cook until the mushrooms are soft, 5 to
   10 minutes. Add the corn and green peas and
   cook for 2 minutes. Add this mixture to the
   potatoes and mix well. Taste and adjust the
   seasoning. Set aside.

3. Preheat the oven to 350°F.

4. To assemble the enchiladas, create a work
   station within easy reach of the stove. Pour
   some enchilada sauce into a shallow dish (to dip
   the tortillas in). Place the filling and the cheese
   close at hand. Spread 1½ cups of the remaining

enchilada sauce into a 9 x 13-inch baking pan that is at least 2 inches deep.

5. Heat a tortilla lightly on a skillet. Dip both sides in the dish of enchilada sauce, and place it in the baking pan. Spoon some of the filling in the center of the tortilla and roll up the tortilla to enclose the filling. Arrange it in the pan seam-side down.

6. Repeat with the remaining tortillas and filling until the pan is filled; make sure to really squeeze them in the pan so that you can fit many of them. Pour some of the remaining enchilada sauce on top; reserve some sauce for serving. Spread or pipe half the cashew cheese over the enchiladas; reserve the remaining cheese.

7. (Alternatively, you can layer the tortillas, filling, and sauce as you would a lasagna, instead of filling each tortilla individually.)

8. Bake until the cheese on top turns a bit brown, about 45 minutes.

9. Serve hot. Pass the reserved warmed enchilada sauce and the remaining cheese at the table, if desired.

THE FORKS OVER KNIVES PLAN

Curried Twice-Baked Potatoes

Makes 8 potato halves

Whenever I bake potatoes—which is often!—I bake a few extra so I have leftovers on hand, ready to make this recipe. Sometimes I even make a double batch of the filling to serve over steamed brown rice—another staple I always have on hand so I can pull together a quick meal. —DS

4 large russet potatoes, scrubbed

Sea salt and freshly ground black pepper

1 medium yellow onion, finely diced

1 medium red bell pepper, seeded and finely diced

2 cloves garlic, minced

1 tablespoon curry powder

1 teaspoon ground coriander

1 teaspoon ground ginger

1 tablespoon arrowroot powder

1 (10-ounce) package frozen spinach

1 cup unsweetened, unflavored plant milk

1. Preheat the oven to 350°F.

2. Wrap each potato in aluminum foil and place them all on a baking sheet. Bake until the potatoes are tender when poked with a sharp knife, about 1 hour. Remove the potatoes from the oven, remove the foil, and let stand until cool enough to handle.

3. When the potatoes are cool, slice them in half lengthwise, gently scoop out the potato flesh, and transfer it to a bowl. Make sure to leave about ½ inch of the flesh in the skin so the halves stay together.

4. Place the potato halves cut-side up on a baking sheet. Lightly season with salt and black pepper. Set aside.

5. Meanwhile, prepare the filling. Place the onion and red bell pepper in a large skillet and cook over medium heat, stirring occasionally and adding water 1 to 2 tablespoons at a time as needed to keep the vegetables from sticking, until the onions start to brown and turn

translucent, 8 to 10 minutes. Add the garlic, curry powder, coriander, and ginger and cook until fragrant, about 1 minute.

6. Add the arrowroot powder, spinach, and plant milk and cook, stirring frequently, until the spinach has thawed and the sauce has thickened, about 3 to 5 minutes. Add the potato flesh to the pan and cook until heated through, breaking up the potato chunks with the side of a wooden spoon. Season to taste with salt and pepper.

7. Spoon the spinach mixture into the potato halves and bake until bubbly, about 30 minutes.

8. Serve hot.

RECIPES

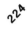
Shepherd's Pot Pie

Makes one (9 × 13-inch) pot pie

A close friend of mine loves to eat my vegetable pot pie with mashed potatoes on top. This recipe is a great way to find out why. —DS

4 large russet potatoes (about 2 pounds), peeled and cut into large chunks

Sea salt

2 large yellow onions, finely diced

3 large carrots, diced

3 cups frozen peas

3 cups frozen corn

4 cups frozen broccoli florets

6 tablespoons arrowroot powder

4 cups unsweetened plant milk

¼ cup nutritional yeast

Freshly ground black pepper

Chopped fresh chives, for serving (optional)

1. Preheat the oven to 350°F.

2. Place the potatoes in a large pot and add water to cover. Bring to a boil over high heat. Reduce the heat to medium, cover the pot, and cook until the potatoes are tender when pierced with the tip of a sharp knife, 12 to 14 minutes. Remove the pot from the heat and drain off all but ⅔ cup of the cooking water. Season the potatoes with salt, and use a potato masher to mash the potatoes well. Set aside.

3. In a large sauté pan, cook the onions and carrots over medium-high heat, stirring occasionally and adding water 1 to 2 tablespoons at a time to keep the vegetables from sticking, until the onions are translucent and beginning to brown, 8 to 10 minutes. Add the peas, corn, and broccoli. Cook until heated through, about 5 minutes.

4. Meanwhile, in a medium bowl, combine the arrowroot powder with the plant milk and whisk until well blended. Add it to the vegetables along with the nutritional yeast and

cook until thickened, about 5 minutes. Season to taste with salt and pepper.

5. Transfer the vegetable mixture to a 9 x 13-inch pan. Spoon the mashed potatoes evenly over the top.

6. Bake until bubbly and lightly browned, about 1 hour. Sprinkle with the chopped chives, if desired, and serve hot.

Quinoa and Sweet Potato Shepherd's Pie

Makes one (9 × 13-inch) shepherd's pie

Shepherd's pie—with its flavorful filling and mashed potato topping—is comfort food at its best. I have several versions that I love; I choose which one to make on any given day depending on my mood and what is in season. This one is a favorite in the fall, which is the natural season for both sweet potatoes and cabbage. —DS

3 large sweet potatoes, peeled and cut into large chunks

1 cup unsweetened, unflavored plant milk

½ teaspoon cayenne pepper (optional)

Sea salt

2½ cups quinoa, rinsed and drained

5 cups vegetable broth, plus more for the vegetables, if desired

1 large yellow onion, diced

2 large carrots, diced

3 cups chopped green cabbage

2 cups frozen peas

2 teaspoons dried thyme

2 teaspoons dried sage, crumbled

1. Preheat the oven to 350°F. Place the sweet potatoes in a large saucepan and add cold water to cover. Bring the water to a boil over high heat. Reduce the heat to low, cover the pan, and cook the sweet potatoes until tender when pierced with the tip of a sharp knife, about 15 minutes.

2. Drain the potatoes and transfer them to a food processor. Add the plant milk and process until pureed. Season with the cayenne pepper (if using) and salt to taste. Set aside.

3. In a large pot, combine the quinoa and vegetable broth and cover with a tight-fitting lid. Bring to a boil over high heat. Reduce the heat to medium-low and cook until the quinoa is tender and the broth has been absorbed, about 15 minutes.

4. While the quinoa is cooking, combine the onion, carrot, and cabbage in a large sauté pan and

cook over medium heat, stirring occasionally and adding water or vegetable broth 1 to 2 tablespoons at a time as needed to keep the vegetables from sticking, until the vegetables are softened and the onions are beginning to brown, about 10 minutes. Add the peas, thyme, and sage and cook just until heated through, about 2 minutes. Stir in the quinoa. Season to taste with salt and pepper.

5. Transfer the quinoa and vegetable mixture to a 9 x 13-inch baking dish and spread it evenly in the pan. Spoon the pureed sweet potatoes over the top and spread it to cover the quinoa.

6. Bake until the top is very lightly browned and bubbling around the edges, about 45 minutes.

7. Serve hot.

Polenta Casserole with Cilantro Chutney

Makes one (8 × 8-inch) casserole

This pie is inspired by dhokla, *one of my favorite traditional dishes that my mother made back in India when I was growing up. It was made of fermented steamed rice cakes and was served with cilantro chutney. I love the chutney because I can add fresh spinach or whatever other greens I have on hand to it and it's always delicious. In fact, I like this chutney so much that some weeks I make it as one of my refrigerator staples to toss with cooked grains or spoon over a baked potato to make a quick and delicious meal.* —DT

Note that you can prepare the pie ahead of time right up through chilling and then bake it just before serving. It's a great main dish but is also a nice appetizer when cut into bite-size squares and served with hot chile sauce (page 272).

FOR THE CILANTRO CHUTNEY

- 1 bunch cilantro, tough stems removed
- 1 bunch spinach, tough stems removed
- ½ cup dried, unsweetened coconut flakes
- ¼ medium onion
- 1 clove garlic
- 3 tablespoons fresh lemon juice (from 1 to 2 lemons)

1. To make the cilantro chutney, rinse the cilantro and spinach well and drain completely, preferably using a salad spinner. Place them in a blender or food processor and add the coconut flakes, onion, garlic, lemon juice, jalapeño, cumin seeds, and salt. Blend together into a paste. Use a rubber spatula to scrape down the sides of the blender, if necessary, but avoid using any added water to create the paste. Set

1 jalapeño, seeded and
  chopped

¼ teaspoon cumin seeds

Sea salt

FOR THE POLENTA

1 teaspoon ground turmeric

¼ teaspoon cumin seeds

Sea salt

1 cup polenta

2 tablespoons fresh lemon
  juice (from 1 lemon)

1 tablespoon sesame seeds

the cilantro chutney aside or transfer to an airtight container and store in the refrigerator for 4 to 5 days.

2. To make the polenta, in a large saucepan, bring 6 cups water to a boil. Add the turmeric, cumin seeds, and salt and cook for 2 minutes.

3. While whisking continuously, add the polenta to the boiling water in a slow and steady stream. Cook over high heat, whisking continuously, for 5 minutes. Stir in the lemon juice. Reduce the heat to maintain a simmer and cook, stirring occasionally, until thick, about 15 minutes.

4. Pour half of the polenta into an 8 x 8-inch baking dish and spread it evenly. Let stand for 10 minutes. (Cover the remaining polenta so that it stays warm and doesn't firm up.)

5. Spread the cilantro chutney over the polenta. Spoon the remaining polenta over the top and spread it gently to completely cover the chutney in an even layer.

6. Sprinkle the sesame seeds over the top. Cover and chill the polenta pie in the refrigerator for 30 minutes.

7. Meanwhile, preheat the oven to 375°F.

8. Bake the polenta until the top of the pie and the sesame seeds are lightly browned, 30 to 45 minutes. Remove from the oven and let the pie stand for a few minutes.

9. Cut into pieces and serve hot.

Roasted Stuffed Winter Squash

Makes 4 stuffed squash halves

Winter squashes, such as acorn and butternut, can be tricky to work with because their tough skin is hard to peel. Preparing squash this way—stuffed with a savory filling and roasted—puts that sturdy shell to good use. The rice should be quite moist after it cooks in step 3; it provides good contrast to the squash and helps the stuffing mixture stay together without becoming chewy or dry during baking. —DT

2 medium acorn squash
½ cup wild rice medley
1 cup low-sodium vegetable broth, plus more as needed
½ medium red onion, finely chopped
1 teaspoon garlic powder
1 teaspoon ground ginger
1½ teaspoons dried rosemary
½ cup finely chopped carrot
½ cup finely chopped red bell pepper
½ cup small broccoli florets
½ cup small cauliflower florets
¼ teaspoon freshly ground black pepper
Sea salt
3 tablespoons pine nuts

1. Cut each acorn squash in half through the stem. Trim the stem and remove and discard the seeds (keep the skin on).

2. Bring a large saucepan or pot of water to a boil. Add the squash halves and cook until the squash is slightly soft when pierced with a fork, 15 to 20 minutes. Remove from the water and drain well. Set aside until cool enough to handle.

3. Meanwhile, bring 1½ cups water to a boil in a small saucepan. Add the wild rice medley and cook, covered, over medium heat for 25 minutes. (Alternatively, follow the cooking instructions on the rice package, using a bit more water than called for so that the rice is moist after steaming.) Remove from the heat and set aside.

4. Use a spoon to scoop out the inner edges of each cooled squash half to create a wider and deeper hollow for the stuffing; leave about half of the squash flesh attached to the peel.

Reserve the scooped-out squash flesh for the stuffing. Set the squash shells aside.

5. Preheat the oven to 350°F.

6. In a skillet with a lid, combine the vegetable broth, onion, garlic powder, ginger, and rosemary. Cover and bring to a boil over high heat. Reduce the heat to medium and cook, covered, until the onion is translucent, about 10 minutes, stirring occasionally.

7. Add the carrot, cover, and cook for about 10 minutes. Add the bell pepper, broccoli, cauliflower, black pepper, and salt to taste, cover, and cook until the vegetables are tender, about 10 minutes more.

8. Add the reserved squash flesh and wild rice. Use a wooden spoon to mix the stuffing together; it should be a bit creamy. If all the liquid has dried up, add about ¼ cup broth or as much as is needed to make it slightly creamy. Taste and adjust the seasoning. Remove from the heat.

9. Arrange the acorn squash shells on a baking sheet and divide the stuffing evenly among them. Sprinkle the pine nuts on top.

10. Bake until the pine nuts are browned and the stuffing is heated through, about 20 minutes. Remove from the oven and let stand for a few minutes before serving. Serve hot.

Polenta Pizza Pie

Makes two (8-inch) pizza pies

*This polenta-based "pizza pie" offers a fresh and delicious
interpretation of both casseroles and pizza! —DT*

FOR THE CRUST

½ teaspoon ground cumin

2 cups polenta

2 tablespoons ground
  flaxseeds

1 teaspoon ground turmeric
  (optional)

Sea salt

FOR THE SAUCE

4 cups finely chopped
  tomatoes

1 cup finely chopped onions

2 cloves garlic

1 teaspoon dried marjoram

1 teaspoon dried thyme

1 teaspoon dried rosemary

1 teaspoon dried oregano

¼ teaspoon ground black
  pepper

½ (6-ounce) can tomato paste

1 tablespoon white wine
  vinegar

Sea salt

1. To prepare the crust, line the sides of two 8-inch round baking pans with strips of parchment paper. Set aside.

2. In a large saucepan, combine 8 cups water with the ground cumin. Bring the water to a boil. While whisking continuously so that it does not form lumps, add the polenta in a slow stream. Add the flaxseed, turmeric (if using), and salt to taste. Cook over medium-high heat until the mixture starts to bubble. Cover the pan, reduce the heat to medium, and simmer until the polenta has soaked up all the water and cooked to a spreadable consistency, 15 to 20 minutes.

3. Divide the polenta evenly between the two prepared pans. Keeping the parchment paper in place, spread the polenta in the pans, making the edges a bit higher than the rest. Let cool to room temperature, and then refrigerate for at least 1 hour. The crust can be prepared a couple of days in advance; if refrigerating for more than an hour, wrap the pans in plastic wrap.

FOR THE TOPPINGS

8 ounces mushrooms, thinly sliced (about 2 cups)

2 medium zucchini, thinly sliced (about 2 cups)

2 medium red bell peppers, finely chopped

¼ cup nutritional yeast, plus more for serving, if desired

¼ cup finely chopped fresh basil

4. To prepare the sauce, in a large saucepan, place the tomatoes, onions, garlic, marjoram, thyme, rosemary, oregano, and black pepper. Cover and cook over medium-low heat for 30 minutes. Add the tomato paste, vinegar, and salt to taste. Cook, uncovered, until the sauce is thickened and the water has evaporated, about 20 minutes. Set aside.

5. To prepare the topping, place the mushrooms in a skillet. Cook over medium heat, uncovered, stirring occasionally, until the mushrooms are soft and the liquid they release is almost completely evaporated, 5 to 7 minutes. Add the zucchini and cook for 5 minutes. Remove from the heat and set aside.

6. In the saucepan cook the bell peppers over medium heat until soft and the liquid released from the bell peppers has evaporated, about 10 minutes. Add the nutritional yeast and cook for 1 minute. Spread the mixture evenly on a small plate, and set aside to cool and allow any remaining moisture to dry. Just before use, mix in the chopped basil.

7. Preheat the oven to 350°F.

8. Remove the baking pans from the refrigerator and let them stand for 20 minutes to bring them to room temperature.

Polenta Pizza Pie *(cont.)*

9. Spread half the pizza sauce on each crust. Spread the mushrooms and zucchini evenly on top. Sprinkle with the bell pepper and basil mixture. Bake until heated all the way through, about 30 minutes.

10. Slice and serve hot. For extra cheesy flavor, sprinkle nutritional yeast on top.

PASTA AND NOODLES

Spaghetti with White Bean Alfredo

Makes about 6 cups

One of the most fat-filled dishes I used to make was pasta with Alfredo sauce. I made it with cream, butter, cheese, and more cheese. This version, on the other hand, is full of flavor without any of the unsavory aftermath of all that fat. —DS

12 ounces whole-grain spaghetti

1 (15-ounce) can navy beans, rinsed and drained

2 tablespoons roasted tahini

2 tablespoons nutritional yeast

1 tablespoon mellow white miso

2 teaspoons fresh lemon juice

2 cloves garlic, chopped

Sea salt and freshly ground black pepper

Chopped fresh parsley, for serving

1. Bring a large pot of water to a boil and cook the spaghetti according to the package instructions. Drain, reserving about ½ cup of the cooking water.

2. Meanwhile, in a blender, combine the beans, tahini, nutritional yeast, miso, lemon juice, and garlic. Puree until smooth and creamy. Add water a little at a time to make a pourable sauce.

3. Transfer the mixture to a saucepan and cook over medium-low heat, stirring frequently, until heated through. Place the sauce in a large bowl, add the cooked pasta to the bowl along with as much of the reserved cooking water as desired to moisten, and toss to coat. Taste and adjust the seasoning. Garnish with chopped parsley. Serve at once.

Sweet Potato Mac and Cheese

Makes about 7 cups

*Sweet potatoes make a surprisingly smooth and creamy sauce
for one of America's favorite dishes. Of course, our version isn't
just delicious; it's also as healthy as it can be! —DS*

1 (14-ounce) box whole-grain macaroni

1 large sweet potato (about 12 ounces), peeled and chopped

1 medium yellow onion, peeled and chopped

½ cup unsweetened, unflavored plant milk, or as needed

½ cup nutritional yeast

2 cloves garlic, minced

½ teaspoon freshly grated nutmeg

½ teaspoon dried rosemary

Sea salt and freshly ground black pepper

1. Preheat the oven to 425°F.

2. Bring a large pot of water to a boil and cook the macaroni according to the package instructions. Drain and transfer the noodles to a large bowl. Set aside.

3. Place the diced sweet potato into a medium saucepan, add water to cover, and bring to a boil. Cook over medium heat until tender when pierced with a sharp knife, 8 to 10 minutes.

4. Drain the potatoes and transfer them to a blender or food processor. Add the yellow onion. Puree until smooth, adding enough plant milk to achieve a creamy texture. Add the nutritional yeast, garlic, nutmeg, rosemary, and salt and pepper to taste. Blend briefly to combine.

5. Pour the sauce over the cooked noodles. Stir until well coated and spoon the mixture into an 8 × 8-inch pan. Bake until the top of the mac and cheese starts to brown, about 15 minutes.

6. Serve hot.

Easy Thai Noodles

Makes about 7 cups

I love Thai food but don't go out to restaurants for it much anymore because it's hard to avoid all the added fat. Here is a quick noodle dish I make about once a week. This one has the great flavor without the fuss or the fat. —DS

8 ounces brown rice noodles or other whole-grain noodles

3 tablespoons low-sodium soy sauce, or to taste

2 tablespoons brown rice syrup or agave nectar

2 tablespoons fresh lime juice (from 1 to 2 limes)

4 cloves garlic, minced

1 (12-ounce) package frozen Asian-style vegetables (about 3 cups)

1 cup mung bean sprouts

2 green onions, white and light green parts chopped

3 tablespoons chopped, roasted, unsalted peanuts

¼ cup chopped fresh cilantro

1 lime, cut into wedges

1. Cook the noodles according to the package instructions. Drain and set aside.

2. Meanwhile in a large saucepan, combine the soy sauce, brown rice syrup, lime juice, garlic, and ¼ cup water. Bring to a boil over medium heat. Stir in the Asian mixed vegetables and cook until crisp-tender, about 5 minutes.

3. Add the cooked noodles and mung bean sprouts and toss to coat. Cook until heated through, about 2 minutes.

4. Garnish the noodles with the green onions, chopped peanuts, cilantro, and lime wedges. Serve.

RECIPES

THE FORKS OVER KNIVES PLAN

Fusilli with Marinara Sauce

Makes about 11 cups

This delicious marinara is so versatile. Use it in your favorite lasagna dish, as a sauce for pizza, tossed with pasta, as we do here, or spooned over a baked potato or polenta. —DS

1 medium yellow onion, finely diced

4 garlic cloves, minced

1 tablespoon tomato paste

1 (28-ounce) can whole peeled Italian tomatoes with their juices, crushed with your hands

½ cup chopped fresh basil

2 teaspoons dried oregano

Sea salt and freshly ground black pepper

1 pound whole-grain fusilli or penne pasta

1. In a large sauté pan, cook the onion over medium heat, stirring occasionally and adding water 1 to 2 tablespoons at a time as needed to keep them from sticking, until translucent and lightly browned, about 10 minutes. Add the garlic and cook for 1 minute. Add the tomato paste and cook for 1 minute. Add the tomatoes, basil, and oregano and cook, uncovered, over medium-low heat until thickened, about 30 minutes.

2. Meanwhile, bring a large pot of water to a boil. When the sauce has about 10 minutes left to cook, prepare the pasta according to the package instructions. Drain, reserving about ½ cup of the cooking water.

3. Transfer the pasta to a large serving bowl. Pour the sauce over the pasta along with as much of the reserved pasta cooking water as desired to moisten and toss well. Taste and adjust the seasoning. Serve hot.

RECIPES

Broccoli Lo Mein

Makes about 6 cups

This dish comes together very quickly once a little chopping is done. In fact, the best way to approach this recipe is to do all the vegetable prep while the water for the linguine is coming to a boil. You can mix up the sauce and stir-fry the vegetables while the noodles cook and the whole dish will come together in minutes after the noodles are done. —DS

12 ounces whole-grain linguine

5 tablespoons low-sodium soy sauce

1½ tablespoons pure maple syrup

1 tablespoon grated peeled fresh ginger

2 cloves garlic, minced

1 medium yellow onion, thinly sliced

3 cups small broccoli florets (from 1 head broccoli)

1. Bring a large pot of water to a boil. Cook the pasta according to the package instructions. Drain and set aside.

2. Meanwhile, in a small bowl, combine the soy sauce, maple syrup, ginger, garlic, and 2 tablespoons water and set aside.

3. Heat a large skillet over high heat. Add the onion and broccoli and cook, stirring occasionally and adding water 1 to 2 tablespoons at a time as needed to keep the vegetables from sticking, until the broccoli is crisp-tender, about 5 minutes.

4. Add the reserved soy sauce mixture and cook for 30 seconds. Add the noodles and toss well. Serve hot.

Spring Thing Pasta

Makes about 13 cups

After a long winter of thick and hearty stews and casseroles, I look forward to cooking with spring's first harvest with bright green flavors. —DS

1 pound whole-grain penne pasta

1 bunch green onions, white and light green parts thinly sliced

1 pound asparagus, trimmed and cut into ½-inch pieces

2 cloves garlic, minced

Sea salt

2 cups shelled fresh or frozen English peas (defrosted, if frozen)

1 cup vegetable broth (optional)

2 teaspoons grated lemon zest

2 teaspoons fresh lemon juice

1 cup chopped mixed herbs, such as parsley, chives, and tarragon

¼ cup pine nuts, toasted (see page 147)

Freshly ground black pepper

1. Bring a large pot of water to a boil. Cook the pasta according to the package instructions. Drain, reserving about 1 cup of the pasta cooking liquid, and set aside.

2. While the pasta is cooking, place a large sauté pan over medium heat. Add the green onions and cook, stirring occasionally and adding water 1 tablespoon at a time to keep the onions from sticking, until softened, about 2 minutes.

3. Add the asparagus, garlic, and salt to taste. Cook, stirring occasionally and adding water as needed to keep from sticking, until the asparagus is tender, about 3 minutes.

4. Stir in the peas and cook for 2 minutes.

5. Add the pasta to the pan along with the reserved pasta cooking water or vegetable broth, if desired. Cook for 2 minutes to heat through.

6. Stir in the lemon zest, lemon juice, herbs, and pine nuts. Season to taste with salt and pepper. Serve hot.

Penne with Tomato-Mushroom Cream Sauce

Makes about 11 cups

Pasta dishes like this one come together easily because I always have most of the ingredients in the pantry and mushrooms in the fridge. If you don't have fresh basil, use 2 tablespoons of dried basil instead. —DS

12 ounces whole-grain penne pasta

1 medium yellow onion, diced

1 pound mushrooms, trimmed and sliced

4 cloves garlic, minced

2 teaspoons dried thyme

1 (28-ounce) can crushed tomatoes, drained

1 cup unsweetened, unflavored plant milk

1 cup chopped fresh basil

Sea salt and freshly ground black pepper

1. Bring a large pot of water to a boil. Cook the pasta according to the package instructions. Drain and set aside.

2. Meanwhile, in a large sauté pan over medium heat, cook the onion and mushrooms, stirring occasionally and adding water 1 to 2 tablespoons at a time as needed to keep the vegetables from sticking, until the onion is translucent and beginning to brown, 7 to 8 minutes.

3. Add the garlic and thyme, and cook for 1 minute. Add the crushed tomatoes and simmer for 10 minutes, stirring occasionally.

4. Add the plant milk, the cooked pasta, the basil, and salt and pepper to taste and toss until well coated. Taste and adjust the seasoning. Cook until heated through, about 1 minute. Serve hot.

RECIPES

Ratatouille Fusilli

Makes about 6 cups

This recipe came about by accident, but it turned out to be such a happy (and delicious) accident that we decided we had to share it. I set about trying to develop a pasta and lentil baked casserole dish, but somewhere between the shopping and the cooking I got off track and came up with this skillet dish instead. The thing is, it's so tasty that Forks Over Knives founder Brian Wendel christened it Ratatouille Fusilli and the rest, as they say, is history. —DT

½ cup green lentils, rinsed and soaked (see page 243)

2 cups fusilli or rotini pasta

1 (15-ounce) can diced tomatoes with their juice

½ cup finely chopped leeks, white and light green parts

1 clove garlic, minced

2¼ teaspoons Italian seasoning

2 small (½ pound) Italian eggplants

½ teaspoon white wine vinegar

2 tablespoons finely chopped fresh basil

1. Place the lentils in a small saucepan and add 1½ cups water. Bring to a boil, then reduce the heat and simmer until the lentils are just cooked, 10 to 15 minutes. Set aside (do not drain).

2. Bring a medium saucepan of water to a boil. Add the pasta and cook according to the package instructions until al dente (avoid overcooking). Drain well and set aside.

3. In a sauté pan, combine the tomatoes with their juice, the leeks, garlic, and Italian seasoning and cook over medium heat for 10 minutes. Stir in the eggplant and cook, partially covered, until the eggplant is completely cooked, stirring occasionally, 15 to 20 minutes.

4. Add the drained pasta, the lentils with their cooking liquid, and the vinegar and toss gently until well combined. Cook until heated through, adding up to ¼ cup water if the mixture seems too dry. Taste and adjust the seasoning. Sprinkle with the basil and serve hot.

Rinsing Grains and Legumes and Soaking Lentils

When our dried ingredients, such as rice and lentils, come in sealed bags, it's easy to forget that they're not that different from fresh vegetables and need to be treated similarly. Place whatever you're rinsing in a large bowl and cover with cold water. Swish it around a few times; the water will often turn creamy white. Drain the water, add fresh water, and repeat 3 or 4 times, or until the water runs clear even after you swish it around. Drain thoroughly before cooking as instructed.

Soaking the lentils for an hour prior to cooking them will reduce the cooking time by 10 to 15 minutes. After soaking, drain them thoroughly and proceed as directed in the recipe, adjusting the cooking time as necessary.

THE FORKS OVER KNIVES PLAN

Spaghetti with Roasted Tomatoes, Chickpeas, and Basil

Makes about 8 cups

Roasting vegetables is an easy way to add flavor to a dish, and, yes, you can absolutely do it without added oil—the results are delectable. —DS

1 pound cherry tomatoes

2 teaspoons granulated garlic

Sea salt and freshly ground black pepper

12 ounces whole-grain spaghetti

1 (15-ounce) can chickpeas, rinsed and drained

1 cup chopped fresh basil

1. Preheat the oven to 350°F. Have a nonstick baking sheet ready or line a regular baking sheet with parchment paper.
2. Bring a large pot of water to a boil.
3. Cut the tomatoes in half and place them in a bowl. Sprinkle them with the granulated garlic and salt and pepper to taste. Spread them on the baking sheet in a single layer. Roast the tomatoes until they start to shrivel, 30 to 35 minutes. Remove from the oven and set aside.
4. During the last 10 minutes that the tomatoes are roasting, add the pasta to the boiling water and cook according to the package instructions. Drain the pasta, reserving about 1 cup of the pasta cooking water. Transfer the pasta to a bowl. Add the chickpeas, the roasted tomatoes, the basil, and as much of the reserved cooking water as desired to moisten, and mix well. Season to taste with salt and pepper. Serve hot.

Quinoa with Red Lentils

Makes about 4 cups

*I enjoy making grain-based dishes like this one because they are
tasty and versatile. I might serve this as a side dish for dinner
one night, and then the next day toss it with greens to make
a hearty salad or eat it all by itself as a meal. —DT*

1 cup red lentils, rinsed and soaked (see page 243)

1 cup finely chopped leek (white and light green parts)

2 cloves garlic, minced

1 tablespoon grated fresh ginger

½ teaspoon chili powder

½ teaspoon ground cumin

1 cup quinoa, rinsed and drained

1 cup yellow bell pepper, cut lengthwise into strips before measuring

1 cup thinly sliced zucchini

1 cup sliced carrots

¼ cup finely chopped cilantro or fresh dill

2 tablespoons fresh lemon juice

Sea salt

1. In a saucepan, place the lentils, leeks, garlic, ginger, chili powder, cumin, and 3 cups water. Bring to a boil over high heat. Reduce the heat to medium, cover the pan, and simmer until the lentils are just slightly tender, 15 to 20 minutes.

2. Add the quinoa, bell pepper, zucchini, carrots, cilantro or dill, lemon juice, and salt to taste. Bring to a boil over high heat. Reduce the heat to low, cover the pan, and simmer until the lentils and quinoa are cooked and the vegetables are tender, about 10 minutes. Taste and adjust the seasoning. Serve hot.

Coconut-Dill Rice

Makes about 6 cups

I find rice so delicious and satisfying that I eat it almost every day. That much rice in my life means that I am always experimenting with new and fun ways to eat it. The beauty of rice is that with just a bit of seasoning and some sliced vegetables, it can be made into a full meal, just as it is here. —DT

1 cup brown rice, rinsed

1 cup thinly sliced onion

½ teaspoon cumin seeds

1 (2-inch) cinnamon stick

4 to 5 small bay leaves

½ yellow bell pepper, seeded and thinly sliced

½ orange bell pepper, seeded and thinly sliced

Sea salt

Pinch of cayenne pepper

¾ cup finely chopped fresh dill

¼ cup dried unsweetened coconut flakes

2 tablespoons fresh lime juice (from 1 to 2 limes)

1. Place the rice in a medium saucepan with 2¼ cups water and bring to a boil. Stir once, reduce the heat to low, cover the pan, and simmer for 45 minutes. Remove from the heat and let stand, covered, for 5 minutes. Remove the cover and fluff with a fork. Set aside.

2. In a skillet with a lid, combine the onion, cumin seeds, cinnamon stick, bay leaves, and ¼ cup water. Cook over high heat, covered, until the onion is softened, about 5 minutes.

3. Add the bell peppers, salt, and cayenne pepper and cook over medium heat, stirring occasionally and adding water 1 to 2 tablespoons at a time as needed to keep the vegetables from sticking, 7 to 10 minutes, until the bell peppers are soft.

4. Add the reserved rice along with the dill, coconut flakes, and lime juice. Stir to blend well. Cook over medium heat until heated through, 3 to 5 minutes. Remove the cinnamon stick and bay leaves. Taste and adjust the seasoning. Serve hot.

RECIPES

Mushroom and Green Pea Risotto

Makes about 6 cups

*This creamy risotto is a vast improvement over the traditional
dish, as it brings all the creamy texture and cheesy flavor
without the heaviness of actual cheese or butter. —DT*

¼ cup cashews

1 cup finely chopped onion

8 ounces button mushrooms,
trimmed and sliced
(2½ cups)

¼ teaspoon freshly ground
black pepper

1 cup fresh or frozen green
peas

6 cups low-sodium vegetable
broth

1 cup short grain brown rice

2 cloves garlic

1 teaspoon dried thyme

1 teaspoon apple cider
vinegar

1 tablespoon nutritional yeast

Sea salt

1. Place the cashews in a small bowl and cover
   with 1 cup water. Set aside to soak for 30
   minutes.

2. In a large skillet with a cover, combine the
   onion and ¼ cup water. Cover and cook over
   high heat for 5 minutes.

3. Stir in the mushrooms and pepper and cook
   over medium heat, uncovered, until the
   mushrooms are tender, 8 to 10 minutes.

4. Add the green peas and cook for 5 minutes,
   adding water 1 to 2 tablespoons at a time as
   needed to keep the vegetables from sticking.
   Remove the pan from the heat and set aside.

5. In a medium saucepan, combine the vegetable
   broth, rice, garlic, and thyme. Bring to a boil
   over high heat. Reduce the heat to medium,
   cover the pan, and simmer, stirring occasionally,
   until the rice is cooked, about 45 minutes.

6. Meanwhile, transfer the cashews and their
   soaking water to a blender. Blend until smooth.
   Set aside.

7. To the pan with the rice add the reserved mushroom mixture and cashew milk along with the vinegar, nutritional yeast, and salt. Cook, uncovered, over medium heat, stirring often, until the rice is completely cooked and still creamy, about 30 minutes (add more water if the liquid has been completely absorbed).

8. Remove the pan from the heat. Cover with a lid and let stand for 5 minutes. Taste and adjust the seasoning. Serve hot.

RECIPES

Polenta Curry

Makes about 6 cups

*Polenta is a satisfying and easy dish to make and its mild flavor
and texture make it a great blank canvas for whatever inspiration
the cook brings to it. In this case, the hearty polenta pairs well
with a rich curry sauce, with truly sublime results. —DT*

FOR THE POLENTA

¼ cup fresh lemon juice
(from 2 or 3 lemons)

1 daikon radish, peeled and
grated

½ teaspoon ground turmeric

½ teaspoon caraway seeds

Sea salt

¾ cup polenta

FOR THE CURRY

4 large tomatoes, cored and
chopped (about 4 cups)

½ large yellow onion, chopped
(about 1 cup)

1 tablespoon raisins

1 tablespoon ground
coriander

1 teaspoon ground cumin

1 teaspoon curry powder

½ teaspoon ground turmeric

⅛ teaspoon cayenne pepper

Sea salt

½ cup frozen green peas

1½ teaspoons fresh lime juice

½ cup finely chopped fresh
cilantro

1. To prepare the polenta, in a large saucepan, bring 5½ cups water to a boil. Add the lemon juice, daikon radish, turmeric, caraway seeds, and a generous pinch of salt and simmer for 2 to 3 minutes.

2. While whisking continuously so that it does not form lumps, add the polenta in a slow stream. Cook on high heat for 5 minutes while continuously stirring with a wooden spoon. Cover and simmer for 10 minutes. Uncover the pan and simmer until the polenta is completely cooked and has the consistency of thick porridge, about 15 minutes.

3. Transfer the polenta to an 8 x 8-inch dish that is at least 1 inch deep. Spread it into an even layer and let it cool to room temperature. Place the dish in the refrigerator for about 30 minutes to set. Remove the dish from the refrigerator. Cut the polenta into 1-inch squares and run a flat spoon or spatula down the lines to thoroughly separate the squares; it is fine to leave them in the dish. Set aside.

RECIPES

4. To prepare the curry, in a blender or food processor, combine the tomatoes, onion, raisins, coriander, cumin, curry, turmeric, cayenne, and salt. Blend until the raisins are well chopped and the mixture is well blended and smooth. Transfer the paste to a skillet and cook over high heat for 15 minutes, stirring occasionally, to cook the tomatoes and onions and allow the spices to blend. Stir in 3 cups water and cook until the sauce thickens slightly and turns a brighter red, about 10 minutes.

5. Add the polenta cubes, green peas, lime juice, and salt to taste. Cook until the sauce thickens, the polenta puffs a bit from absorbing the sauce, and the peas are cooked through, 5 to 10 minutes; do not overcook or the polenta will fall apart. Taste and adjust the seasoning. Garnish with cilantro and serve hot.

THE FORKS OVER KNIVES PLAN

Rye and Wheat Berries with Celery and Apples

Makes about 6 cups

I love this refreshing summer salad just as it is presented here, but it can easily be adapted to accommodate what's in season or what's in your pantry and refrigerator. Switch up the grains, fruit, and herbs—try barley in place of one of the grains here along with pears and cilantro, for instance—and you'll have an entirely different result that is just as easy to put together and equally delectable. —DT

¼ cup wheat berries

¼ cup rye berries

3 tablespoons fresh lemon juice (from 1 to 2 lemons)

⅛ teaspoon cayenne pepper

⅛ teaspoon ground cumin

Sea salt

3 stalks celery, cut into 1-inch pieces

2 sweet, juicy apples, such as Gala or Fuji, cored and cut into 1-inch pieces

¾ cup finely chopped fresh parsley

¼ cup golden raisins

1. In a small bowl, combine the wheat and rye berries and add water to cover generously. Set aside to soak for 2 hours. Drain and transfer to a small saucepan. Add 3 cups water and bring to a boil over high heat. Reduce the heat to medium, and cook, covered, until the berries are soft to the bite, about 30 minutes. Drain and set aside to cool.

2. In a small bowl, whisk together the lemon juice, cayenne, cumin, and salt to taste. Set aside.

3. Place the cooled berries in a large bowl. Add the celery, apples, parsley, raisins, and lemon juice mixture. Toss gently until well combined. Taste and adjust the seasoning. Serve at room temperature or chilled. Store in an airtight container in the refrigerator for up to 3 days.

RECIPES

Millet in Coconut Curry

Makes about 6 cups

I'm always looking for new ways to serve millet, which is fabulously versatile but can be tricky to prepare. Here's a delicious and foolproof way to serve it: in a bursting-with-flavor coconut curry. —DT

¾ cup millet

1 medium leek, white and light green parts finely chopped (about 1 cup)

2 cloves garlic, minced

1½ tablespoons grated peeled fresh ginger

4 or 5 bay leaves

1 bunch asparagus, cut into 1-inch pieces (about 2 cups)

1 (15-ounce) can light coconut milk

1 date, pitted and finely chopped

⅛ teaspoon freshly ground white or black pepper

Sea salt

1 tablespoon fresh lime juice, or as needed

2 tablespoons finely chopped fresh cilantro

1. In a small saucepan, bring 2½ cups water to a boil. Add the millet, reduce the heat to low, cover the pan, and simmer for 10 minutes (all of the water will not be absorbed). Remove the pan from the heat and set aside, covered, for at least 10 minutes.

2. In a sauté pan, combine the leek, garlic, ginger, and bay leaves with ½ cup water. Cook over medium heat, stirring occasionally, for 5 minutes. Add the asparagus and cook until the liquid has evaporated and the asparagus is crisp-tender, 8 to 10 minutes.

3. Add the millet along with the coconut milk, date, pepper, and salt to taste. Cook over medium-high heat until the milk comes to a boil. Remove and discard the bay leaves. Stir in the lime juice. Taste and add more salt or lime juice as needed. Garnish with the cilantro and serve hot.

RECIPES

Quinoa and Millet with Kale and Roasted Butternut Squash

Makes about 8 cups

This is a great lunch or dinner dish no matter what season it is. During the summer, serve it chilled on a bed of greens, and during the winter, serve it at room temperature with a cup of hot soup. —DT

1 small butternut or acorn squash (about 1 pound)

3 cups stemmed and finely chopped kale

½ cup finely chopped fresh parsley

¼ cup fresh lemon juice (from 2 to 3 lemons)

1 small clove garlic, minced

Sea salt and freshly ground black pepper

½ cup quinoa

½ cup millet

⅓ cup slivered almonds

¼ cup raisins

1. Preheat the oven to 375°F. Cut the squash in half and scoop out and discard the seeds. Place the squash skin-side up on a rimmed baking sheet and bake until tender, 50 to 60 minutes. Set aside until completely cool. Peel off the skin and cut the squash into ½-inch cubes.

2. Meanwhile, in a large bowl, combine the kale, parsley, lemon juice, garlic, and salt and pepper to taste. Let stand for 30 minutes.

3. In a small saucepan, bring 2 cups water to a boil. Add the quinoa and millet and return to a boil. Reduce the heat to low, cover the pan, and simmer for 10 minutes. Remove from the heat and let stand, covered, for at least 10 minutes. When the liquid is absorbed, remove the cover and let cool.

4. While the grains cook, place the almonds in a medium skillet and toast over medium-low heat, stirring frequently, until lightly browned and fragrant, 5 to 7 minutes. Immediately transfer the nuts to a plate to cool.

5. Add the squash, quinoa-millet, and raisins to the kale mixture. Stir gently to combine. Taste and adjust the seasonings. Top with the toasted almonds. Serve at room temperature or chilled.

RECIPES

RECIPES

Easy Veggie Stir-Fry

Makes about 3 cups

*When your grain of the week is in the fridge and you have a package
or two of frozen vegetables in the freezer, dinner can be blissfully
uncomplicated to pull together—and tasty, too! —DS*

2 cloves garlic, minced

1 teaspoon grated peeled fresh ginger

1 tablespoon low-sodium soy sauce

1 tablespoon brown rice syrup

1 medium yellow onion, diced

1 (12-ounce) package frozen Asian-style vegetables (about 3 cups)

2 cups cooked brown rice (see page 181)

1. In a small bowl, combine the garlic, ginger, soy sauce, and brown rice syrup. Stir until well blended and set aside.

2. Heat a skillet over medium-high heat. Add the onion and cook, stirring occasionally and adding water 1 to 2 tablespoons at a time as needed to keep the onions from sticking, for 3 minutes.

3. Add the frozen vegetables and the soy sauce mixture. Cook, stirring frequently, until the vegetables are heated through, 5 to 7 minutes. Serve hot over brown rice.

Red Beans and Quinoa

Makes about 10 cups

I've had a version of beans and rice on my dinner menu for as long as I can remember, mostly because it's always tasty and filling, and I can make it as easy or as complicated as I want it to be. This version is definitely on the easier side of the scale, as I've switched out the rice for delicious quinoa, a good stand-in for rice because it has nice texture, good grassy flavor, and, best of all, it can be cooked very quickly. This is an ideal weeknight meal or weekend brunch dish. —DS

1 large onion, chopped

1 green bell pepper, seeded and chopped

2 stalks celery, chopped

2 tablespoons minced garlic

1 tablespoon dried thyme

3 (15-ounce) cans kidney beans, rinsed and drained

4 cups vegetable broth

2 cups quinoa, rinsed

Sea salt and freshly ground black pepper

1 teaspoon red pepper flakes, or to taste (optional)

1. Place the onion, bell pepper, and celery in a large saucepan over medium-high heat. Cook, stirring occasionally and adding water 1 to 2 tablespoons at a time as needed to keep the vegetables from sticking, until the onions start to turn translucent, about 5 minutes.

2. Add the garlic and thyme and cook until the garlic is softened and fragrant, about 1 minute. Add the kidney beans and vegetable broth. Bring to a boil over medium-high heat. Reduce the heat to medium-low and cook, covered, to allow the flavors to come together, about 10 minutes.

3. Stir in the quinoa. Season with salt, black pepper, and red pepper flakes (if using), and simmer, covered, until the quinoa is cooked and the flavors are well blended, 12 to 15 minutes. Taste and adjust the seasoning. Serve hot.

RECIPES

SAUCES, DIPS, DRESSINGS, AND SALSAS

Red Beet Dip

Makes about 1 cup

When I first served this to my guests, the idea of a dip made with red beets didn't sound appealing to them. But once they tried it, they could not stop eating it! This dip tastes even better the next day, which makes it especially nice for a gathering for which you want to do some preparation ahead of time. Serve it with sliced vegetables, crackers, or chips. —DT

¼ cup cashews

1 medium red beet, peeled, trimmed, and cut into 1-inch pieces

1 clove garlic

¼ cup finely chopped red onion

3 tablespoons very finely chopped fresh flat-leaf parsley

1 teaspoon Dijon mustard

Sea salt

Pinch of freshly ground black pepper

Raw vegetables, crackers, or baked tortilla chips, for serving

1. Place the cashews in a small bowl and cover with at least ½ cup water. Set aside to soak for about 45 minutes. Drain thoroughly.

2. Meanwhile, bring a small saucepan of water to a boil. Add the beet and simmer until very tender when poked with a fork, 25 to 30 minutes. Drain and let stand until completely cool.

3. Transfer the cooled beet to a blender or food processor along with the drained cashews and the garlic. Blend into a paste.

4. Transfer to a bowl and add the onion, parsley, mustard, salt to taste, and pepper. Stir until well combined. Place in the refrigerator until well chilled, 1 to 2 hours. For longer storage, store in an airtight container for 4 to 5 days.

5. Serve with raw vegetables, crackers, or tortilla chips for dipping.

Artichoke Dip

Makes about 2½ cups

*This dip is easy to prepare at the last minute as a great appetizer
or snack served on crackers or whole-grain crostini. —DS*

1 (15-ounce) can low-sodium cannellini or other white beans, rinsed and drained

¼ cup pine nuts, toasted (see page 147)

2 tablespoons drained capers

1 tablespoon dried basil

1 (15-ounce) can artichoke hearts packed in water, drained

Sea salt and freshly ground black pepper

1. In a food processor, combine the beans, pine nuts, capers, and basil. Process until smooth and creamy. (The mixture may be very thick, which is fine.)

2. Add the artichoke hearts and pulse 5 or 6 times until they are partially chopped; you want some of the artichoke hearts to still be intact. Season to taste with salt and pepper.

3. Serve immediately or store in an airtight container in the refrigerator for up to 4 days.

RECIPES

White Bean and Rosemary Spread

Makes about 1¼ cups

*I always have some kind of bean spread on hand in my fridge. I like to
eat them in wraps, dip veggies in them, or use them as a sauce on pizza.
I love how easy it is to make this one—so I make it a lot. —DS*

1 (15-ounce) can white beans,
such as cannellini, navy, or
great northern, rinsed and
drained

3 tablespoons roughly
chopped shallot

2 cloves garlic

1 tablespoon balsamic vinegar

1 teaspoon ground rosemary

½ teaspoon freshly ground
black pepper

Sea salt

1. In a food processor, combine the beans, shallot,
garlic, vinegar, rosemary, pepper, and a pinch of
salt. Process until smooth and creamy. Taste and
adjust the seasoning as necessary.

2. Serve at room temperature. Store in an airtight
container in the refrigerator for up to 1 week.

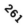
Lentil-Pecan Hummus

Makes about 1¾ cups

I created this hummus one day while trying to devise a good use for leftover lentils. I also had some toasted pecans left over from a salad I'd made, so I put them together and voilà! Success! I love to eat this in a whole-grain wrap with sprouts and grated carrots. —DS

⅔ cup green lentils, rinsed

⅓ cup pecans, toasted (see page 147)

3 cloves garlic

2 tablespoons fresh lemon juice (from about 1 lemon)

1 teaspoon ground cumin

Sea salt

Pinch of cayenne pepper

1. Place the lentils in a small saucepan and add water to cover. Bring to a boil over high heat, then reduce the heat to medium and simmer until the lentils are very tender, 20 to 30 minutes, adding water as necessary to keep the lentils covered. Drain (you should have 2 cups lentils). Set aside to cool completely.

2. In a food processor, combine the lentils, pecans, garlic, lemon juice, cumin, salt to taste, and cayenne. Process until smooth and creamy.

3. The hummus is best served at room temperature. Store in an airtight container in the refrigerator for up to 1 week.

Sun-Dried Tomato Hummus

Makes about 3 cups

This is a tangy and very flavorful hummus with a lovely burnt-orange color. The chickpeas need to soak for 1 to 6 hours, so be sure to plan ahead if using dried chickpeas. —DT

1 cup dried chickpeas, soaked (see page 160)

¾ cup sun-dried tomatoes (not packed in oil)

3 tablespoons fresh lime juice (from about 2 limes)

1 clove garlic

¼ to ½ teaspoon freshly ground black pepper

Sea salt

Sliced vegetables, for serving

1. Place the soaked chickpeas in a medium saucepan with 4 cups water. Bring the water to a boil, then reduce the heat to medium and simmer until the chickpeas are very soft, 40 to 50 minutes. Remove from the heat and set aside to cool to room temperature; do not drain.

2. Meanwhile, place the sun-dried tomatoes in a small bowl and pour 1 cup warm water over them. Let stand until softened, about 30 minutes. Drain well and transfer to a blender or food processor.

3. Add the cooled chickpeas and their cooking liquid along with the lime juice, garlic, pepper, and salt to taste. Blend into a smooth paste, adding water as needed to reach the desired consistency. Taste and adjust the seasoning. Cover and chill until ready to serve, or, for longer storage, transfer the hummus to an airtight container and store in the refrigerator for 4 to 5 days.

4. Serve chilled or at room temperature with assorted sliced vegetables.

Sun-Dried Tomato Tapenade

Makes about 1½ cups

*I love this tapenade as a topping for baked potatoes, or tossed
with warm pasta for a quick, flavorful meal. —DS*

**4 ounces sun-dried tomatoes
(not packed in oil)**

¼ cup drained capers

1 clove garlic, minced

**3 fresh basil leaves, roughly
chopped**

Zest of 1 lemon

1. Place the sun-dried tomatoes in a medium bowl
   and add warm water to cover. Let stand until
   softened, about 15 minutes. Drain well.

2. Transfer the drained tomatoes to a food
   processor and add the capers, garlic, basil, and
   lemon zest. Process until the mixture becomes a
   chunky paste. Serve immediately or refrigerate
   until ready to use. Store in an airtight container
   in the refrigerator for up to 1 week.

RECIPES

Ginger-Miso Sauce

Makes about ½ cup

*I love this sauce for its versatility—as delicious on steamed
vegetables and brown rice as it is as a marinade for tofu. —DS*

⅓ cup rice vinegar

2 tablespoons mellow white miso

1 tablespoon chopped peeled fresh ginger

2 large cloves garlic

1. In a blender, combine the vinegar, miso, ginger, and garlic. Blend until smooth and creamy. Add up to ¼ cup water as needed to achieve a creamy consistency.

2. Use immediately or store in an airtight container in the refrigerator for up to 1 week.

Wasabi Orange Sauce

Makes about 1½ cups

*This sauce is a very good salad dressing, and I often make a double batch so I
have enough for the rolls and can save the rest to make tossed salads. —DT*

3 medium oranges, peeled and seeded

2 small dates, pitted

3 tablespoons peanut butter

2¼ teaspoons low-sodium tamari

¾ teaspoon prepared wasabi paste

1. Place the oranges, date, peanut butter, tamari, and wasabi paste in a blender or food processor and blend until smooth.

2. Transfer to a bowl, cover, and chill for 30 minutes before serving. The dressing will keep in an airtight container in the refrigerator for 4 to 5 days. Serve cold.

Creamy Herbed Salad Dressing

Makes about 3 cups

This dressing is great on just about any salad and also makes a creamy topping for baked potatoes or a great dip for a fresh vegetable tray (cut back on the added water if using as a dip). —DS

1 (12-ounce) package extra-firm silken tofu

½ cup red wine vinegar

½ cup fresh basil, roughly chopped

1½ tablespoons roughly chopped fresh tarragon or 2 teaspoons dried tarragon

3 cloves garlic

½ teaspoon sea salt

Freshly ground black pepper

1. In a blender, combine the tofu, vinegar, basil, tarragon, garlic, salt, and ½ cup water. Blend until smooth and creamy. Add pepper to taste.
2. Use immediately or store in an airtight container in the refrigerator for up to 1 week.

Creamy Poppy Seed Dressing

Makes about 2 cups

I often toss this on salad, but my hands-down favorite use for it is as a dressing for coleslaw. —DS

1 (12-ounce) package firm silken tofu

¼ cup agave nectar or brown rice syrup

¼ cup rice vinegar

2 tablespoons poppy seeds

1 tablespoon Dijon mustard

1 teaspoon onion powder

½ teaspoon sea salt

1. In a blender, combine the tofu, agave, vinegar, poppy seeds, mustard, onion powder, and salt. Blend until smooth and creamy.
2. Use immediately or store in an airtight container in the refrigerator for up to 7 days.

RECIPES

Cucumber-Tahini Dressing

Makes about 1½ cups

*This dressing lends itself to hearty lettuces, such as romaine,
or to being tossed with shredded Napa cabbage for an unusual
twist on classic coleslaw. Its cool and nutty flavor is also welcome
drizzled over steamed vegetables and brown rice. —DS*

1 medium cucumber, peeled,
seeded, and chopped

⅓ cup roasted tahini

¼ cup fresh lemon juice
(from about 2 lemons)

2 cloves garlic

½ teaspoon sea salt, or to
taste

Pinch of cayenne pepper
(optional)

1. In a blender, combine the cucumber, tahini, lemon juice, garlic, salt, and cayenne (if using). Process until smooth and creamy. Add water a little at a time as needed to achieve a pourable consistency. Taste and adjust the seasoning as desired.

2. Use immediately or store in an airtight container in the refrigerator for up to 7 days.

Raspberry Vinaigrette

Makes about 1½ cups

I make a lot of this zesty dressing in the summer when raspberries are fresh at the farmers' market. It's very good on spicy greens like arugula. I eat it on anything, including a spoon. It is refreshing and light, and delicious. —DS

2 cups raspberries, rinsed

4 teaspoons balsamic vinegar

3 tablespoons roughly chopped shallot

2 tablespoons brown rice syrup

1½ teaspoons dried tarragon

½ teaspoon sea salt, or to taste

Freshly ground black pepper

1. In a blender, combine the raspberries, balsamic vinegar, shallot, brown rice syrup, tarragon, salt (if using), and pepper to taste. Blend until smooth and creamy with a pourable consistency. If necessary, add water 1 tablespoon at a time and blend briefly after each addition to achieve the desired consistency.

2. Use immediately or store in an airtight container in the refrigerator for up to 7 days.

RECIPES

Creamy Tomato-Basil Dressing

Makes about 2 cups

This dressing is just the thing to pull together a delicious salad of pasta, chopped fresh zucchini, red bell pepper, and thinly sliced red onion. —DS

1 large ripe tomato, cored and chopped

1 cup roughly chopped fresh basil

½ cup rinsed and drained cooked or canned white, cannellini, pinto, or navy beans

6 tablespoons red wine vinegar

1 tablespoon Dijon mustard

3 cloves garlic

Sea salt and freshly ground black pepper

1. In a blender, combine the tomato, basil, beans, vinegar, mustard, and garlic. Blend until smooth and creamy, adding up to ½ cup water. Taste and add salt and pepper as needed.

2. Use immediately or store in an airtight container in the refrigerator for up to 5 days.

Balsamic Vinaigrette

Makes about 1¼ cups

This is a perfect pantry dressing—use it as your go-to for your favorite salad or as a marinade for grilled or roasted vegetables. —DS

1 cup balsamic vinegar
¼ cup brown rice syrup
2 tablespoons Dijon mustard
3 tablespoons roughly chopped shallot
Freshly ground black pepper

1. In a small bowl, whisk together the vinegar, brown rice syrup, mustard, shallot, and pepper to taste.
2. Use immediately or store in an airtight container in the refrigerator for up to 1 week.

Sour "Cream"

Makes about 1½ cups

This is delicious on top of Corn and Black Bean Cakes (page 142), as well as on steamed vegetables; lentil soup; and, naturally, steamed or baked potatoes. —DS

1 (12-ounce) package firm or extra-firm silken tofu
3 tablespoons white wine vinegar
Sea salt

1. Combine the tofu and vinegar in a food processor and process until smooth and creamy. Add salt to taste.
2. Use immediately or store in an airtight container in the refrigerator for up to 1 week.

RECIPES

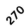

Del's Basic Barbecue Sauce

Makes about 2¾ cups

Barbecue sauce is not just for pork or chicken! I make baked beans and sloppy joes with it, and even use it as a sauce for grilled portobello mushrooms. —DS

1 medium onion, minced

1 clove garlic, minced

1 cup tomato sauce

¼ cup apple cider vinegar, plus more as needed

3 tablespoons vegan Worcestershire sauce, or 2 tablespoons low-sodium soy sauce

2 tablespoons maple syrup

2 tablespoons unsulphured molasses

3 tablespoons prepared yellow mustard

Freshly ground black pepper

1. In a large saucepan, cook the onion over medium heat, stirring occasionally and adding water 1 to 2 tablespoons at a time as needed to keep it from sticking, until translucent and starting to brown, 7 to 8 minutes. Add the garlic and cook for another minute.

2. Stir in the tomato sauce, vinegar, Worcestershire sauce, maple syrup, molasses, mustard, pepper to taste, and 1 cup water and bring to a boil over high heat. Reduce the heat to low and simmer, stirring often to prevent scorching, until thickened, about 45 minutes. Taste and adjust the seasoning. If desired, use an immersion blender or transfer to a blender to blend the sauce until smooth.

3. Store in an airtight container in the refrigerator for up to 7 days.

Enchilada Sauce

Makes about 9 cups

This tangy sauce is exactly what you need to prepare Potato Enchiladas (page 220) or a South-of-the-Border Pizza (page 163). And when there's some on hand in the refrigerator, a very quick meal can be made by stirring some sauce into a pot of rice, beans, and sautéed onions and peppers. —DT

1 large yellow onion, roughly chopped

3 pounds tomatoes, cored and roughly chopped

1 (6-ounce) can tomato paste

3 cloves garlic

1 tablespoon ground cumin

2 tablespoons sweet paprika

¼ teaspoon smoked hot paprika

1 tablespoon onion powder

1½ teaspoons garlic powder

1½ teaspoons dried oregano

Sea salt

½ teaspoon arrowroot powder

1. In a blender or food processor, combine the onion, tomatoes, tomato paste, and garlic. Blend until smooth. (Do this in batches if necessary.) Transfer to a saucepan and stir in the cumin, paprika, onion powder, garlic powder, oregano, a generous pinch of salt, and 3 cups water. Bring to a boil over medium heat and cook for 10 to 15 minutes.

2. Meanwhile, in a small bowl, mix the arrowroot powder with 1 tablespoon water, stirring well to avoid any lumps. Add this to the sauce, stirring well. Simmer, covered, for 15 to 20 minutes, until the sauce reduces a bit and is fragrant. Taste and adjust the seasoning.

3. Store in an airtight container in the refrigerator for up to 7 days.

RECIPES

Hot Chile Sauce

Makes about 1 cup

I created this sauce when I could not easily find a commercially made hot sauce that was oil- and sugar-free—and also tasted really good! Plus, I really wanted to control the heat to my personal preference. This delicious sauce meets all my specifications. It also stays fresh in the fridge for a good long time, so I can make a batch and keep it awhile. I call that an all-around winner! —DT

1 red bell pepper

2 ripe medium tomatoes, cored and quartered

2 tablespoons onion powder

1 tablespoon garlic powder

⅛ teaspoon cayenne pepper, or to taste

⅛ teaspoon apple cider vinegar

Sea salt

1½ teaspoons arrowroot powder

1. Place the whole bell pepper in a dry skillet and roast over medium-high heat, turning the pepper often to cook all sides, until it is charred and wilted all over, 10 to 15 minutes. Alternatively, roast the pepper in a preheated 375°F oven for about 30 minutes.

2. Remove the pepper from the skillet or oven and wrap it in a clean kitchen towel. Let it cool for 15 to 20 minutes. Unwrap the towel, and peel off the charred skin. Cut the pepper in half and remove and discard the seeds and core.

3. Transfer the pepper to a blender or food processor. Add the tomatoes, onion powder, garlic powder, cayenne pepper, vinegar, and salt to taste. Blend until smooth.

4. Transfer to a medium saucepan and bring to a boil over medium-high heat. Simmer, uncovered, stirring occasionally, until the sauce is very fragrant and slightly thickened, 15 to 20 minutes.

5. Meanwhile, in a small bowl mix the arrowroot

powder with ½ cup water and stir until smooth. Stir the mixture into the sauce. Cook until the sauce has thickened and is a translucent glaze, 10 to 15 minutes.

6. Meanwhile, bring a saucepan of water to a rolling boil. Place a 12-ounce glass jar in the water and boil gently for 5 minutes. Remove to a drying rack and let air dry. If the lid is metal, it can also be dipped in the boiling water for 30 seconds and set aside to air dry. (If the lid is plastic, run it through the dishwasher.)

7. When the sauce is done, remove the pan from the heat and let it sit for a moment. Pour the sauce into the sterilized jar while the sauce is still hot, leaving some headspace at the top. Close with the sterilized lid. Let cool completely at room temperature.

8. Make sure the jar is tightly closed. Store in the refrigerator; the sauce will be good for at least 1 month.

Tomato Salsa

Makes about 1 cup

A friend of mine taught me his family recipe for salsa roja de molcajete, *or tomato salsa made in a traditional stone mortar and pestle. I've adapted it so that I can make it without the* molcajete. *Roasting the chile and the tomatoes brings out the authentic earthy taste even without the traditional tools.* —DT

1 (2-inch) piece dried red
   chile, any hot variety
6 ripe plum tomatoes
2 (½-inch-thick) onion wedges
1 clove garlic
Sea salt
1 tablespoon finely chopped
   fresh cilantro

1. Place the dried chile in a skillet and cook over high heat for 1 to 2 minutes until the chile puffs up or gets some dark spots; be careful not to burn the chile or it will be bitter. Remove the chile from the pan and set aside to cool.

2. Place the whole tomatoes in the skillet and roast over medium heat. Turn them periodically as they get charred and roast until almost the entire surface is charred, about 10 minutes. Remove the tomatoes from the heat and set aside to cool.

3. Place 2 of the tomatoes in a blender along with the roasted chile, the onions, garlic, and salt to taste. Blend into a smooth sauce. Add the remaining tomatoes and pulse so that the salsa is well blended but still chunky. Stir in the cilantro. Taste and adjust the seasoning. Transfer to a bowl, cover, and chill until ready to serve. For longer storage, transfer to an airtight container and store in the refrigerator for 4 to 5 days.

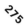

DESSERTS

Chocolate Raspberry Parfaits

Makes 6 parfaits

*Chocolate and raspberries have a natural affinity for each other,
as is well showcased in this delicious dessert. —DS*

FOR THE RASPBERRY CREAM

2 cups fresh raspberries

3 tablespoons pure maple
syrup

1 (12-ounce) package firm
silken tofu

1 tablespoon fresh lemon juice

FOR THE CHOCOLATE CREAM

1 (12-ounce) package firm
silken tofu

⅓ cup unsweetened cocoa

¼ cup pure maple syrup

½ teaspoon pure vanilla
extract

¼ teaspoon sea salt

½ cup fresh raspberries, for
garnish

1. To make the raspberry cream, in a small
saucepan, combine the raspberries and maple
syrup. Cook over medium-low heat until the
raspberries start to break down, about 10
minutes. Transfer the mixture to a blender.
Add the tofu and lemon juice and blend until
smooth and creamy. Transfer to a bowl, cover,
and refrigerate the mixture until completely
cool.

2. To make the chocolate cream, place the tofu,
cocoa, maple syrup, vanilla, and salt in a
blender. Puree until smooth and creamy.

3. To serve, fill 6 (6-ounce) parfait cups halfway
with the chocolate cream. Fill the ramekins the
remainder of the way with the raspberry cream.

4. Chill for 1 hour before serving. The chocolate
and raspberry layers can be made separately
1 day ahead and then assembled to serve.

5. Just before serving, garnish each ramekin with
a few of the fresh raspberries.

RECIPES

THE FORKS OVER KNIVES PLAN

Fudgy Brownies

Makes 12 brownies

Every now and then I want something chocolaty, and these brownies do the trick every time. They are moist and rich and full of melt-in-your-mouth chocolate flavor. Yum! —DS

¾ cup pure maple syrup

½ cup unsweetened applesauce

1 egg replacer egg (I use Ener-G Egg replacer)

1 teaspoon pure vanilla extract

⅓ cup unsweetened cocoa powder

½ cup whole-grain spelt flour

½ cup finely chopped walnuts (optional)

¼ teaspoon aluminum-free baking powder

¼ teaspoon baking soda

¼ teaspoon sea salt

1. Preheat the oven to 350°F. Line an 8-inch square pan with parchment paper.

2. In a medium bowl, combine the maple syrup, applesauce, egg replacer, and vanilla and whisk until well blended.

3. In a large bowl, whisk together the cocoa powder, spelt flour, walnuts, baking powder, baking soda, and salt.

4. Add the maple syrup mixture to the flour mixture and gently fold them together with a rubber or wooden spatula.

5. Spread the batter into the prepared pan and bake until the top of the brownie block is firm to the touch, about 30 minutes.

6. Place the pan on a wire rack to cool for 1 hour. Use the parchment to pick up the brownie block and transfer it to a cutting board. Slice into 12 squares; for clean cuts, wipe the knife after each cut and dip in hot water. Store the brownies in an airtight container in a cool place for 3 to 4 days.

RECIPES

Chewy Lemon-Oatmeal Cookies

Makes 14 to 16 cookies

*The trick to keeping these chewy, flavorful cookies moist is the
low-and-slow baking—45 minutes at 275°F—which allows
them to bake through without drying out. —DT*

10 dates, pitted

1 cup unsweetened
applesauce

1½ teaspoons apple cider
vinegar

1 cup rolled oats

1 cup oat flour

½ cup quick-cooking oats

¾ cup roughly chopped
walnuts

2 tablespoons grated lemon
zest (from about 2 lemons)

2 teaspoons natural cocoa
powder

1 teaspoon vanilla powder

½ teaspoon baking soda

Pinch of sea salt

1. Preheat the oven to 275°F. Line 2 baking sheets
   with parchment paper.

2. Place the dates in a medium bowl and
   cover with hot water. Set aside to soak for
   20 minutes. Drain any excess water from the
   bowl and transfer the dates to a blender or food
   processor. Add the applesauce and vinegar and
   blend into a paste. Set aside.

3. In a large bowl, stir together the rolled oats, oat
   flour, quick-cooking oats, walnuts, lemon zest,
   cocoa powder, vanilla powder, baking soda, and
   salt. Add the date and applesauce paste and
   use a wooden spoon to mix lightly but well. The
   mixture should be on the dry side.

4. Scoop a golf-ball-size portion of dough with
   your hands. Gently roll it into a ball and then
   pat it flat; be very gentle and do not compact it.
   Place the round on the prepared baking sheet
   and repeat with the remaining dough.

5. Bake until the tops of the cookies appear crispy
   and browned, 35 to 45 minutes. Transfer to a
   wire rack to cool. Store in an airtight container
   at room temperature for 4 to 5 days (if they last
   that long without being gobbled up!).

No-Bake Peanut Wonders

Makes 18 to 20 cookies

I always make some variation of these cookies for the holidays. The beauty of this recipe is that you can replace up to 1 cup of the dates with any dried fruit and use different nuts to create your own version of this cookie. Feel free to play around and come up with your own favorite version! —DS

2 cups chopped pitted dates

2 cups roasted, unsalted, no-oil-added peanuts, plus 1 cup ground peanuts, for rolling

2 tablespoons unsweetened cocoa powder (optional)

½ teaspoon pure vanilla extract

Pinch of sea salt

1. In a food processor, combine the dates, the 2 cups whole peanuts, the cocoa powder (if using), the vanilla, and the salt. Process until mostly smooth—when you squeeze the mixture in your hands, it should hold together.

2. Place the 1 cup ground peanuts in a small dish.

3. Using a small cookie scoop or a tablespoon, scoop up the dough and use your hands to shape it into a ball. Roll the ball in the ground peanuts until completely coated. If the peanuts do not easily adhere to the ball, moisten the ball with a little bit of water, either by brushing it with water or by wetting your hands and rolling the ball in them before coating it with the peanuts. Continue with the remaining dough and ground peanuts.

4. Store in an airtight container at room temperature for up to 5 days.

RECIPES

Carrot Cupcakes

Makes 12 cupcakes

These moist cupcakes have a special-occasion flair about them, but the real beauty here is that they can be made entirely from pantry and crisper-drawer staples! —DT

FOR THE CUPCAKES

2 cups whole wheat flour or gluten-free sorghum flour

½ teaspoon ground cardamom

¼ teaspoon baking soda

2 teaspoons baking powder

2 pinches of salt

¾ cup unsweetened, unflavored plant milk

¾ cup pure maple syrup

½ cup unsweetened applesauce

1 teaspoon apple cider vinegar

1 cup grated carrots

1 tablespoon ground flaxseeds

FOR THE FROSTING

¾ cup cashews

2 cups grated carrots

½ cup pure maple syrup

Pinch of sea salt

2 tablespoons slivered almonds, toasted (see page 147), for decoration (optional)

1. Preheat the oven to 350°F. Line a standard 12-cup muffin tray with paper cupcake liners.

2. In a large bowl, whisk together the flour, cardamom, baking soda, baking powder, and salt. Set aside.

3. In a medium bowl, whisk together the plant milk, maple syrup, applesauce, and vinegar. Add the carrots and flaxseeds and stir until well combined.

4. Gently stir the milk mixture into the flour mixture. Pour the batter into the muffin tray, dividing it evenly among the 12 cups.

5. Bake until a toothpick inserted in the center of a cupcake comes out clean, about 25 minutes.

6. Remove from the oven and let the cupcakes cool in the pan for a few minutes. Transfer the cupcakes to a wire rack to cool to room temperature.

7. Meanwhile prepare the frosting. Place the cashews in a small bowl and add at least 1 cup

water. Set aside to soak for 1 hour. Drain and set aside.

8. In a small saucepan, combine the carrots and ½ cup water. Cook over high heat, covered, until all the water has evaporated, about 10 minutes. Add the maple syrup and cook, uncovered, until the maple syrup is absorbed by the carrots and glazes them, 2 to 3 minutes. Remove from the heat and let cool for 5 minutes.

9. Transfer the carrots and syrup to a blender. Add the reserved cashews and salt. Blend until smooth; do not add water or any other liquid. Transfer to a bowl, cover, and chill until needed. For longer storage, transfer the frosting to an airtight container and store in the refrigerator for 2 to 3 days.

10. Use a small spatula to coat the top of each cupcake with some of the frosting. Sprinkle with the almonds and serve. Store the cupcakes in a covered container at room temperature for 2 to 3 days.

Rice Pudding with Mixed Berry Sauce

Makes 6 puddings

*Chia seeds undergo a remarkable transformation when soaked in water—
they plump up and develop a jellylike coating, making them a wonderful
textural addition to all sorts of dishes. If you have clear pudding cups
or even cocktail glasses, these puddings make a beautiful presentation
as you can see the layers of pudding, chia seeds, and deep purple-red
berry sauce. Even in opaque ramekins, the layers present to lovely
effect when you taste it, with creamy pudding, gelled yet crunchy chia
seeds, and sweet-tart berry sauce combining with each bite. —DT*

**FOR THE MIXED BERRY
SAUCE**

10 ounces strawberries,
hulled (2 cups)

1 cup blueberries

1 cup raspberries

2 tablespoons pure maple
syrup

½ teaspoon arrowroot powder

FOR THE RICE PUDDING

3 tablespoons chia seeds

1 tablespoon pure maple syrup

½ cup brown rice flour

8 dates, pitted and chopped

½ cup unsweetened
applesauce

1½ teaspoons vanilla powder

½ teaspoon apple cider
vinegar

⅛ teaspoon ground cinnamon

6 to 12 walnut pieces, for
serving (optional)

1. To prepare the mixed berry sauce, place the
   strawberries, blueberries, raspberries, maple
   syrup, and arrowroot powder in a blender
   or food processor. Blend until pureed, then
   transfer the mixture to a small saucepan.

2. Cook over medium heat until the sauce comes
   to a boil and thickens a bit, 4 to 5 minutes.
   Remove from the heat and transfer to a bowl.
   Let cool completely. For longer storage, transfer
   the sauce to an airtight container and store in
   the refrigerator for up to 1 week.

3. To prepare the rice pudding, place the chia
   seeds in a small bowl with 1 cup water and
   ½ tablespoon of the maple syrup. Set aside until
   the water has been absorbed and the seeds are
   gelatinous, 1 to 2 hours.

4. In a large saucepan, bring 5 cups water to a
   boil. While whisking continuously so that it

does not form lumps, add the brown rice flour in a slow stream. Add the dates and cook over medium heat, whisking occasionally, until the mixture comes to a boil.

5. Stir in the remaining ½ tablespoon maple syrup along with the applesauce, vanilla powder, vinegar, and cinnamon. Simmer, stirring continuously, until the mixture thickens, about 20 minutes. If there are any lumps or if the dates are not completely cooked into the sauce, transfer to a blender or use an immersion blender to blend into a consistent creamy texture.

6. Divide the rice pudding evenly among 6 (10-ounce) clear ramekins or pudding cups. Place the ramekins on a small baking sheet and set in the freezer for 15 minutes.

7. Remove the ramekins from the freezer. Sprinkle about 2 tablespoons of the chia seeds on top of each and spread gently to cover the surface.

8. Place the ramekins back in the freezer until the top layer is set firm, about 20 minutes.

9. Remove the ramekins from the freezer and pour 2 to 3 tablespoons of the mixed berry sauce on top of each. Place in the refrigerator until ready to serve, or store, covered, for 3 or 4 days. Just before serving, place 1 or 2 walnut pieces on top of each pudding. Serve cold.

284

Banana Mango Ice "Cream"

Makes about 1 quart

One of the most satisfying desserts (or anytime sweet treats) I make is also one of the simplest. Freezing fresh fruit and then processing it in a blender until smooth and creamy makes delicious ice "cream." Here are two of my favorite combinations, presented as a main recipe and variation. Let your imagination (and the season) dictate which combinations you prepare. The very best and creamiest results will be achieved if you use a Champion juicer or Vitamix-style high-performance blender. You can certainly use a regular blender or food processor and will have very good results; it may be necessary to add a little bit of water and let the fruit soften a few minutes. After years of using my regular blender I finally treated myself to a more powerful tool (in my case, the Champion), just to make ice creams like these. I've been thoroughly enjoying the fantastic results it yields ever since! —DT

4 ripe bananas
2 ripe mangoes

1. Peel the bananas. Peel the mangoes and cut the flesh from the pit. Place the bananas and mango flesh on a baking sheet or in another flat container, making sure not to pile the fruits too close to each other. Place in the freezer until completely frozen, at least 2 to 3 hours. Also place an empty 2-quart container in the freezer.

2. To prepare the ice "cream," place the frozen bananas in a blender (or juicer) and pulse until blended into a creamy paste. Add water a few drops at a time if necessary to keep the fruit moving, and if the blades are not catching the

fruit, let it stand at room temperature for a few minutes to soften it slightly.

3. Transfer the pureed bananas to the chilled container. Place the frozen mangoes in the blender (or juicer) and blend to a creamy texture. Transfer to the container with the bananas.

4. Quickly yet gently stir the two purees together; do not worry if they are not completely blended. Work quickly so the ice "cream" does not melt into a liquid.

5. Serve at once or store in the freezer for 1 or 2 days, until ready to serve. Remove from the freezer 20 to 25 minutes before serving to soften.

Apple and Fig Ice "Cream"

Makes about 1 quart

2 apples, peeled, cored, and quartered

8 ripe figs, trimmed

Proceed as directed for Banana Mango Ice "Cream," pureeing half the fruits at a time and then gently combining them.

RECIPES

Banana Ice "Cream" with Chocolate Sauce

Makes about 1 quart and about 1 cup sauce

FOR THE CHOCOLATE SAUCE

½ cup cashews

¼ cup pure maple syrup

1 tablespoon unsweetened cocoa powder

1 teaspoon vanilla powder

Pinch of sea salt

FOR THE BANANA ICE "CREAM"

6 ripe bananas

2 tablespoons slivered almonds, toasted (see page 147), for serving

1. To prepare the chocolate sauce, place the cashews in a small bowl and add at least ¾ cup water. Set aside to soak for 1 hour. Drain the cashews and transfer to a blender. Add the maple syrup, cocoa powder, vanilla powder, and salt. Blend until smooth, adding ¼ cup water a few drops at a time as needed to keep the mixture moving in the blender. Transfer to a bowl and set aside until needed. For longer storage, transfer the sauce to an airtight container and store in the refrigerator for up to 3 days. Bring to room temperature before using.

2. To make the banana ice "cream," proceed as directed for Banana Mango Ice "Cream" (on page 284) pureeing half of the bananas at a time and then gently combining them.

3. Toast the almonds in a skillet over medium heat until lightly browned and fragrant, 5 to 7 minutes. Transfer to a plate to stop the cooking and set aside to cool.

4. To serve, scoop some ice "cream" into a bowl, pour the chocolate sauce over the top, and sprinkle with the toasted almonds.

Apple Crisp

Makes 3 to 4 cups

There's something about the fall that makes apple crisp seem so right, but I'm just as happy with this crisp when I replace the apples with peaches or pears. Feel free to do the same and substitute your own favorite fruit for the apples. —DS

FOR THE FILLING

7 medium Granny Smith apples, cored and thinly sliced (about 8 cups)

¾ cup cane sugar

½ teaspoon ground cinnamon

¼ teaspoon freshly grated nutmeg

2 tablespoons whole wheat pastry flour

FOR THE TOPPING

¾ cup rolled oats

¼ cup whole wheat pastry flour

¼ cup cane sugar

½ teaspoon ground cinnamon

⅓ cup unsweetened applesauce

1. Preheat the oven to 375°F.

2. To prepare the filling, combine the apples, sugar, cinnamon, and nutmeg and toss until well coated. Transfer the apples to a large saucepan or Dutch oven. Cook over low heat until the apples start to release their juices, about 5 minutes. Sprinkle the flour over the apple mixture and cook until the filling thickens, about 5 minutes. Transfer the mixture to an 8 x 8-inch baking dish and set aside.

3. To prepare the topping, in a medium bowl, whisk together the oats, flour, sugar, and cinnamon. Add the applesauce and stir to blend. Scatter the mixture over the apples in the baking dish.

4. Cover the dish with foil and bake for 40 minutes. Remove the foil and bake until the filling starts to bubble, about 15 minutes more. Serve hot or warm.

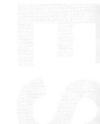

Acknowledgments

We would like to thank our families for their continued support and belief in us. Thanks to Brian Wendel and the Forks Over Knives team for giving us this amazing opportunity and for helping us with it every step of the way. We thank Marah Stets for working her magic and translating our thoughts to print. Thank you, Del Sroufe and Darshana Thacker, for making living this way easy, exciting, and delicious. Thanks to Michelle Howry and the team at Touchstone for bringing this message to life and for making it available to so many people. And, finally, we give our heartfelt thanks to John McDougall for teaching us to practice medicine this way.

WEEK 1 (BREAKFAST)

HOW DOES THIS MEAL PLAN WORK?

We want you to be in control of what you eat, when you eat, and how much you eat. In the long run, this freedom from specific "diets" and "plans" will be liberating. However we know that in the short term, adopting a whole-food, plant-based diet can seem like navigating a brand-new and unfamiliar city without a map of any kind. So if you would like more structure, especially at the beginning of your transition, we offer here a transition plan—based on the information and recipes in this book, *The Forks Over Knives Plan*—that will help you move effortlessly from your current diet to a whole-food, plant-based one in four weeks.

Although we suggest a specific meal plan for each day (this week, you're only changing each day's breakfast), it's important that you remember your own needs—including how much time you have available for shopping and cooking as well as your personal preferences. Feel free to switch around or swap out recipes to meet those needs. For your convenience, after each recipe you will find the recipe's page number and approximate preparation time.

HOW TO SAVE TIME ON COOKING AND PREP

Whenever possible plan ahead. Read through the recipe when you make your shopping list, and the night before to make sure you have all the ingredients and any substitutes you would like to use. Some dishes may require prep work such as chopping vegetables and soaking grains or beans. Do whatever prep work you can the night before to save time in the morning. And take a few minutes to lay out your tools (measuring cups and spoons, mixing utensils, saucepans, etc.). This is especially helpful when you are trying out a new recipe or for a dish that takes longer than a few minutes to prepare.

WHAT TO DO WITH LEFTOVERS

Some days you will have leftovers from the previous day's breakfast. You can enjoy it again just as is the next morning, or you can change the way you serve it. For example, spoon some different fresh fruit over the Multigrain Pancakes; sprinkle nuts on top of the Breakfast Fruit Crisp; serve the Twice Baked Sweet Potatoes on toast; or make a sandwich out of leftover Potato Scramble.

If you don't have enough leftovers to make a complete breakfast, bulk it up by adding any of the following quick options: fruit salad; quick-cooking oatmeal; a smoothie; or a sandwich or wrap made with a nut butter and sliced fruit.

A NOTE ON YIELDS

Most of our recipes yield enough for 4 to 5 people. The following recipes are exceptions and need to be scaled up as indicated to accommodate this many people:

- The Easiest Granola: 2 times
- Fruit & Nut Oatmeal: 2 times
- Breakfast Smoothie: 2 times
- The Quickest Breakfast Wrap: 4 times

If you are cooking for more or fewer people, scale the recipes up or down accordingly.

We often quote Dr. Caldwell B. Esselstyn, Jr. who likes to say that people choosing a whole-food, plant-based lifestyle become "the locus of control" of their own health and vitality. This week, by taking the relatively small step of changing just one meal each day, you are taking a giant leap toward your own empowerment. Now let's leap right into Week One's plan!

WEEK 1 AT A GLANCE

	Breakfast	Lunch	Dinner	Dessert
Day 1	**THE EASIEST GRANOLA** With plant-based milk and fresh fruit Make 2 times the recipe Page 144 (60 minutes)			

*Tip: We suggest **The Easiest Granola** as the first meal of the plan, as it can be made in advance (it'll keep for up to 10 days), and it is good for those mornings when you don't have the time to prepare something fresh. This granola also makes a good snack any time of the day. If you are making it for a family, or you want to have lots on hand this week for yourself, we recommend that you double the recipe.*

	Breakfast	Lunch	Dinner	Dessert
Day 2	**THE QUICKEST BREAKFAST WRAP** Make 4 times the recipe Page 145 (2 minutes) or **LEFTOVERS FROM DAY 1**			

*Tip: If you are gluten-free, substitute corn tortillas for the **Breakfast Wrap**.*

	Breakfast	Lunch	Dinner	Dessert
Day 3	**BAKED BREAKFAST POLENTA WITH BERRY COMPOTE** Page 153 (15 minutes) or **LEFTOVERS FROM DAY 2**			

*Tip: If you are having the **Breakfast Wrap** again, try it on toasted bread instead of rolled into a tortilla.*

	Breakfast	Lunch	Dinner	Dessert
Day 4	**FRUIT AND NUT OATMEAL** Make 2 times the recipe Page 152 (10 minutes) or **LEFTOVERS FROM DAY 3**			

*Tip: If you like a crunchier flavor, try steel-cut oats instead of the rolled oats in the **Fruit and Nut Oatmeal**.*

	Breakfast	Lunch	Dinner	Dessert
Day 5	**BIG BREAKFAST BURRITO** Page 151 (50 minutes) **TOMATO SALSA** Page 274 (15 minutes) or **LEFTOVERS FROM DAY 4**			

*Tip: If preparing the **Tomato Salsa** yourself, you can make it up to 4 or 5 days in advance. Or use store-bought, to save time.*

	Breakfast	Lunch	Dinner	Dessert
Day 6	**BREAKFAST SMOOTHIE** Make 2 times the recipe Page 148 (3 minutes) or **LEFTOVERS FROM DAY 5**			

Tip: If you are having a smoothie for breakfast, plan to eat an extra snack or a bigger lunch today, as you may find you are hungrier earlier.

	Breakfast	Lunch	Dinner	Dessert
Day 7	**POTATO SCRAMBLE** on whole-wheat bread or tortillas Page 150 (35 minutes) or **LEFTOVERS FROM DAY 6**			

*Tip: You can make the scramble up to 2 days in advance to save time this morning. Eat any leftover potato scramble for lunch tomorrow, when we suggest you have it with the **Beet and Barley Salad**. Or you can have it for breakfast tomorrow. If you want a little variety, eat it in a wrap tomorrow if you have it on toast today.*

WEEK 2 (BREAKFAST AND LUNCH)

WHAT'S NEW THIS WEEK?

Congratulations on completing Week 1! We hope you are enjoying your transition and finding some meals that you will be able to enjoy for years to come. In this week, we will be keeping breakfast and adding lunch to your meal plan.

HOW TO SAVE TIME ON COOKING BREAKFAST AND LUNCH

As we suggested earlier, planning goes a long way, so whenever possible take time to plan out your lunch for the following day. For example, the Potato Scramble you had for breakfast yesterday will make a great lunch today. You can bulk up any lunch by adding some extra salad, brown rice, or a dip on the side. Cooking beans and grains takes a little more time, so try setting aside some time over the weekend to prepare a variety of beans and grains to use during the week. You can even pack some of these into the freezer so you'll always have some on hand.

WHAT TO DO WITH LEFTOVERS

Leftovers can now work for both breakfast and lunch. Save cooking time by eating them the following day, or freeze them and save them for later. Leftovers can also be used with your evening meals, even if they are not yet plant based. You may even find that with so many leftovers you don't need to cook as often. If you are choosing to eat leftovers the following day, stave off boredom by adding a side dish or two, such as a salad, grain of the week, or soup to freshen things up.

WEEK 2 AT A GLANCE

	Breakfast	Lunch	Dinner	Dessert
Day 8	**THE QUICKEST BREAKFAST WRAP** Page 145 (2 minutes) or **LEFTOVERS FROM DAY 7**	**BEET AND BARLEY SALAD** Page 176 (40 minutes, plus soaking time for the barley) with **LEFTOVER POTATO SCRAMBLE FROM DAY 7**		

*Tip: For the **Beet and Barley Salad**, soak the barley at breakfast time. Or, if you are going to prepare the lunch in the morning, soak it the previous night. Cook the beets at the same time.*

	Breakfast	Lunch	Dinner	Dessert
Day 9	**MULTIGRAIN PAN-CAKES WITH FRESH BERRIES** Page 141 (45 minutes) or **LEFTOVERS FROM DAY 8**	**CREAM OF BROCCOLI SOUP** Page 201 (30 minutes) with **WHITE BEAN AND ROSEMARY SPREAD** Page 260 (5 minutes) with whole-grain pita bread or lettuce leaves or **LEFTOVERS FROM DAY 8**		

Tip: You can make the **Multigrain Pancakes** in half the time if you use two nonstick pans or a large griddle, so that you can cook more pancakes at a time. If you have any leftover pancakes, you can store them in the fridge and reheat for breakfast tomorrow.

	Breakfast	Lunch	Dinner	Dessert
Day 10	**FRUIT AND NUT OATMEAL** Make 2 times the recipe Page 152 (10 minutes) or **LEFTOVERS FROM DAY 9**	**SLOPPY JOE PITAS** Page 156 (35 minutes) **DEL'S BASIC BARBECUE SAUCE** Page 270 (55 minutes) or **LEFTOVERS FROM DAY 9**		

Tip: Make the **Barbecue Sauce** up to 7 days before or use store-bought.

	Breakfast	Lunch	Dinner	Dessert
Day 11	**CORN AND BLACK BEAN CAKES** Page 142 (50 minutes) **TOMATO SALSA** Page 274 (15 minutes) **SOUR "CREAM"** Page 269 (2 minutes) or **LEFTOVERS FROM DAY 10**	**NO-FUSS PASTA SALAD** Page 179 (20 minutes) **BALSAMIC VINAIGRETTE** Page 269 (2 minutes) or **LEFTOVERS FROM DAY 10**		

Tip: Make the **Tomato Salsa** up to 4 or 5 days in advance, or use store-bought. For the **No-Fuss Pasta Salad**, you can use any leftover vegetables. You can also use store-bought balsamic vinaigrette.

	Breakfast	Lunch	Dinner	Dessert
Day 12	**BREAKFAST SMOOTHIE** Make 2 times the recipe Page 148 (2 minutes) or **LEFTOVERS FROM DAY 11**	**SPINACH-POTATO TACOS** Page 170 (35 minutes) or **LEFTOVERS FROM DAY 11**		

	Breakfast	Lunch	Dinner	Dessert
Day 13	**TWICE-BAKED BREAKFAST SWEET POTATOES** Page 146 (90 minutes) or **LEFTOVERS FROM DAY 12**	**MIXED BEAN AND VEGETABLE STEW** Page 190 (70 minutes) **BROWN RICE** Make 3 times the recipe Page 181 (60 minutes) or **LEFTOVERS FROM DAY 12**		

Tip: If making rice, make 3 times the recipe and freeze the extra rice in two two separate portions for Days 15 and 18.

	Breakfast	Lunch	Dinner	Dessert
Day 14	**THE EASIEST GRANOLA** Make 2 times the recipe Page 144 (60 minutes) or **LEFTOVERS FROM DAY 13**	**PASTA E FAGIOLI** Page 212 (30 minutes) Fresh green salad with **RASPBERRY VINAIGRETTE** Make 2 times the recipe Page 267 (2 minutes) or **LEFTOVERS FROM DAY 13**		

Tip: *Make an extra portion of the* **Raspberry Vinaigrette** *for Day 16.*

WEEK 3 (BREAKFAST, LUNCH, AND DINNER)

WHAT'S NEW THIS WEEK?

By now you might already be a pro at preparing the meals, knowing how to substitute ingredients, and creating fresh new dishes out of leftovers. These will be great tools to incorporate as we add dinner to the meal plan this week.

HOW TO SAVE TIME

Presoaking or prepping the night before or the day of can help save a lot of time, as can appliances like an electric Crock-Pot, rice cooker, or pressure cooker for preparing grains, legumes, and beans—just set the timer and let them take care of the rest!

WEEK 3 AT A GLANCE

	Breakfast	Lunch	Dinner	Dessert
Day 15	**BREAKFAST FRUIT CRISP** Page 149 (50 minutes) or **LEFTOVERS FROM DAY 14**	**HOLLYWOOD BOWL BROWN RICE SALAD** Page 189 (35 minutes, using **BROWN RICE LEFT OVER FROM DAY 13** if desired) or **LEFTOVERS FROM DAY 14**	**LIMA BEAN SOUP** Page 205 (40 minutes) **SHEPHERD'S POT PIE** Page 224 (85 minutes) **LEFTOVERS FROM DAY 14**	**FRESH OR FROZEN FRUIT**

Tip: **The Hollywood Bowl Brown Rice Salad** *will taste as good with any other grain. Throw in some cooked beans to make it even heartier.*

	Breakfast	Lunch	Dinner	Dessert
Day 16	**BAKED BREAKFAST POLENTA WITH BERRY COMPOTE** Page 153 (15 minutes) or **LEFTOVERS FROM DAY 15**	**BLACK-EYED PEA BURGERS** Page 154 (105 minutes) Fresh green salad with **RASPBERRY VINAIGRETTE LEFT OVER FROM DAY 14** or **LEFTOVERS FROM DAY 15**	**PENNE WITH TOMATO-MUSHROOM CREAM SAUCE** Page 241 (25 minutes) or **LEFTOVERS FROM DAY 15**	**FRESH OR FROZEN FRUIT**

Tip: *You can make a double batch of the* **Black-Eyed Pea Burgers** *and enjoy in the following days.*

	Breakfast	Lunch	Dinner	Dessert
Day 17	**THE QUICKEST BREAKFAST WRAP** Make 4 times the recipe Page 145 (2 minutes) or **LEFTOVERS FROM DAY 16**	**RYE AND WHEAT BERRIES WITH CELERY AND APPLES** Page 252 (40 minutes, plus soaking time for rye and wheat berries) or **LEFTOVERS FROM DAY 16**	**TEX-MEX BEAN AND CORNBREAD CASSEROLE** Page 219 (60 minutes) or **LEFTOVERS FROM DAY 16**	**BANANA MANGO ICE "CREAM"** Page 284 (15 minutes, plus 2 to 3 hours freezing time)

Tip: *For the* **Rye and Wheat Berries,** *soak the grains the previous night. Also, you can change the grains and fruits to your preference. Add some beans to make this a heartier meal.*

	Breakfast	Lunch	Dinner	Dessert
Day 18	**MULTIGRAIN PANCAKES WITH FRESH BERRIES** Page 141 (45 minutes) or **LEFTOVERS FROM DAY 17**	**SHIITAKE MUSHROOM LETTUCE WRAP** Page 162 (20 minutes) **BROWN RICE LEFT OVER FROM DAY 13** or **LEFTOVERS FROM DAY 17**	**LENTIL-VEGETABLE STEW** Page 194 (107 minutes) Steamed quinoa Fresh green salad with **CREAMY HERBED SALAD DRESSING** Page 265 (2 minutes) or **LEFTOVERS FROM DAY 17**	**FRESH OR FROZEN FRUIT**

Tip: The **Lentil-Vegetable Stew** will work with any grain, so pick your favorite.

	Breakfast	Lunch	Dinner	Dessert
Day 19	**POTATO SCRAMBLE** on whole-wheat bread or tortillas Page 150 (35 minutes) or **LEFTOVERS FROM DAY 18**	**CREAMY SPINACH SOUP** with toasted multigrain bread Page 200 (35 minutes) with **WHITE BEAN LETTUCE WRAP** Page 161 (10 minutes) or **LEFTOVERS FROM DAY 18**	**FUSILLI with MARINARA SAUCE** Page 238 (50 minutes) or **LEFTOVERS FROM DAY 18**	**FRESH OR FROZEN FRUIT**

Tip: Frozen ripe bananas make a delicious dessert. Peel them before freezing and store in containers. Have them plain or with some jam or nut butter.

	Breakfast	Lunch	Dinner	Dessert
Day 20	**FRUIT AND NUT OATMEAL** Make 2 times the recipe Page 152 (10 minutes) or **LEFTOVERS FROM DAY 19**	**ASIAN WRAP** Page 172 (45 minutes) or **WASABI ORANGE SAUCE** Page 264 (2 minutes) or **LEFTOVERS FROM DAY 19**	**POLENTA PIZZA PIE** Page 232 (140 minutes) Fresh green salad with **CREAMY TOMATO-BASIL DRESSING** Page 268 (2 minutes) or **LEFTOVERS FROM DAY 19**	**NO-BAKE PEANUT WONDERS** Page 279 (20 minutes)

Tip: You can prep the ingredients for the **Asian Wrap** and make the **Wasabi Orange Sauce** beforehand. You can use the leftover sauce as a dressing over salad. To save time with the **Polenta Pizza**, make the crust earlier in the day and let it chill in the fridge.

	Breakfast	Lunch	Dinner	Dessert
Day 21	**BIG BREAKFAST BURRITO** Page 151 (50 minutes) **TOMATO SALSA** Page 274 (15 minutes) or **LEFTOVERS FROM DAY 20**	**JAMAICAN FRUITED RICE SALAD** Page 175 (65 minutes) with **BROWN RICE** Page 181 (60 minutes) or **LEFTOVERS FROM DAY 20**	**ROASTED STUFFED WINTER SQUASH** Page 230 (60 minutes) **BORSCHT (BEET SOUP)** Page 193 (50 minutes) or **LEFTOVERS FROM DAY 20**	**FRESH OR FROZEN FRUIT**

Tip: If preparing the **Tomato Salsa** yourself, make it up to 4 or 5 days in advance. Or use store-bought to save time. Make 2 batches of brown rice to be used in the following days. Using leftover rice, or any other precooked grain, with the **Jamaican Fruited Rice Salad** will cut the cooking time to 20 minutes.

WEEK 4 (BREAKFAST, LUNCH, AND DINNER)

WHAT'S NEW THIS WEEK?

Actually, we're not making any big changes to your meal plan this week, as you've been eating three full whole-food, plant-based meals since last week. This week you want to cement your transition so it will last a lifetime. Use this week to clean up around the edges. If you've been hanging on to a few animal-based products either at a meal or in a snack here and there, actively look for whole-food, plant-based alternatives this week. As you head into this week, consider whether there were any times of day last week that you felt like you were missing or craving something. Here again, actively seek out healthy alternatives, and if you found that you were hungry at unexpected times last week, eat more this week! By the end of the next seven days, you will have completed your Forks Over Knives transition. Then there will be nothing more to do than enjoy your newfound vitality and good health. Cheers to you!

WEEK 4 AT A GLANCE

	Breakfast	Lunch	Dinner	Dessert
Day 22	**BREAKFAST SMOOTHIE** Make 2 times the recipe Page 148 (2 minutes) or **LEFTOVERS FROM DAY 21**	**30-MINUTE CHILI** Page 192 (30 minutes) Whole-grain noodles or **LEFTOVERS FROM DAY 21**	**POTATO-VEGETABLE CHOWDER** Page 204 (45 minutes) Spinach or any other greens with **CUCUMBER-TAHINI DRESSING** Page 266 (2 minutes) or **LEFTOVERS FROM DAY 21**	**FRESH OR FROZEN FRUIT**

Tip: Bake a big batch of potatoes in the oven at 400 degrees for 40–50 minutes. Keep some in the fridge to supplement other meals or as a snack.

	Breakfast	Lunch	Dinner	Dessert
Day 23	**CORN AND BLACK BEAN CAKES** Page 142 (50 minutes) **TOMATO SALSA** Page 274 (15 minutes) **SOUR "CREAM"** Page 269 (2 minutes) or **LEFTOVERS FROM DAY 22**	**RED BEET DIP** Page 258 (47 minutes) with toasted whole-grain pita Fresh green salad with **BALSAMIC VINAIGRETTE** Make 2 times the recipe Page 269 (2 minutes) or **LEFTOVERS FROM DAY 22**	**RICE CASSEROLE WITH LENTILS AND SAUTÉED VEGETABLES** Page 216 (65 minutes) Sautéed kale or Swiss chard **LEFTOVERS FROM DAY 22**	**CHOCOLATE RASPBERRY PARFAIT** Page 275 (20 minutes)

*Tip: Make extra **Balsamic Vinaigrette** for dinner on Day 25. If preparing the **Tomato Salsa** yourself, make it up to 4 or 5 days in advance. Or use store-bought to save time.*

	Breakfast	Lunch	Dinner	Dessert
Day 24	**BREAKFAST FRUIT CRISP** Page 149 (50 minutes) or **LEFTOVERS FROM DAY 23**	**NAVY BEAN HUMMUS AND MIXED VEGETABLE PITA POCKETS** Page 168 (45 minutes) or **LEFTOVERS FROM DAY 23**	**TORTILLA SOUP** Page 206 (45 minutes) **SOUTH-OF-THE-BOR-DER PIZZA** Page 163 (25 minutes) or **LEFTOVERS FROM DAY 23**	**FRESH OR FROZEN FRUIT**

*Tip: Pick your favorite vegetables and mix it up to get new flavors for your **Pita Pockets**.*

	Breakfast	Lunch	Dinner	Dessert
Day 25	BAKED BREAKFAST POLENTA WITH BERRY COMPOTE Page 153 (15 minutes) or LEFTOVERS FROM DAY 24	QUINOA WITH RED LENTILS served on a bed of greens or kale Page 245 (40 minutes) or LEFTOVERS FROM DAY 24	SWEET POTATO LASAGNA Page 213 (40 minutes) or BALSAMIC VINAIGRETTE LEFT OVER FROM DAY 23 or LEFTOVERS FROM DAY 24	FRESH OR FROZEN FRUIT

	Breakfast	Lunch	Dinner	Dessert
Day 26	TWICE-BAKED BREAKFAST SWEET POTATOES Page 146 (90 minutes) or LEFTOVERS FROM DAY 25	BUTTERNUT SQUASH SOUP WITH GREEN PEAS AND PESTO SAUCE Page 202 (35 minutes) Leftover bread or grains or LEFTOVERS FROM DAY 25	SPAGHETTI WITH WHITE BEAN ALFREDO Page 235 (25 minutes) Steamed vegetables with CREAMY HERBED DRESSING Page 265 (2 minutes) or LEFTOVERS FROM DAY 25	CHEWY LEMON-OATMEAL COOKIES Page 278 (80 minutes)

Tip: Add any leftover grains like rice or quinoa, or a salad to your lunch to bulk it up.

	Breakfast	Lunch	Dinner	Dessert
Day 27	THE QUICKEST BREAKFAST WRAP Make 4 times the recipe Page 145 (2 minutes) or LEFTOVERS FROM DAY 26	BLACK BEAN AND RICE BURRITO Page 158 (75 minutes) or LEFTOVERS FROM DAY 26	PIZZA WITH CREAMED SPINACH, SUN-DRIED TOMATOES, RED ONION, AND OLIVES Page 164 (45 mins) MASHED POTATOES AND GRAVY Page 180 (80 minutes) or LEFTOVERS FROM DAY 26	FRESH OR FROZEN FRUIT

Tip: Add some greens to your **Mashed Potatoes** to pack an even greater nutrient punch!

	Breakfast	Lunch	Dinner	Dessert
Day 28	THE EASIEST GRA-NOLA Make 2 times the recipe Page 144 (60 minutes) or LEFTOVERS FROM DAY 27	MILLET CROQUETTES WITH DILL DIPPING SAUCE Page 182 (90 minutes) served over a bed of salad greens or lettuce leaves or LEFTOVERS FROM DAY 27	CHICKPEA CHILI ON BAKED POTATOES Page 210 (65 minutes) or LEFTOVERS FROM DAY 27	FRESH OR FROZEN FRUIT

Tip: To mix things up, **Chickpea Chili** can also be poured over leftover grains or baked sweet potatoes. Or, if eating pizza left over from yesterday, reheat it in a 400°F oven for 5 to 10 minutes. Line the baking tray with parchment paper to prevent the crust from getting soggy.

Resources

TO LEARN MORE

For more information, or to become actively involved in the field of plant-based nutrition, check out these websites:

- Dr. McDougall's Health and Medical Center: www.drmcdougall.com
- Engine 2 Diet: www.engine2diet.com
- Engine 2 Retreats: www.engine2retreats.com
- Forks Over Knives: www.forksoverknives.com
- Happy Cow, the Healthy Eating Guide: www.happycow.net
- Jeff Novick, MS, RD: www.JeffNovick.com
- Physicians Committee for Responsible Medicine: www.pcrm.org
- Prevent and Reverse Heart Disease: www.heartattackproof.com
- T. Colin Campbell Center for Nutrition Studies: www.nutritionstudies.org
- TrueNorth Health Center: www.healthpromoting.com
- Wellness Forum: www.wellnessforum.com

BOOKSHELF

Following are some essential books for the plant-based bibliophile:

- *21-Day Weight-Loss Kickstart,* by Neal D. Barnard, MD, Grand Central, 2011.
- *Bravo!: Health-Promoting Meals from the TrueNorth Kitchen,* by Ramses Bravo, Book Publishing Company, 2012.
- *Breaking the Food Seduction,* by Neal D. Barnard, MD, St. Martin's Press, 2003.

- *Chef Del's Better Than Vegan*, by Del Sroufe with Glen Merzer, BenBella Books, 2013.

- *Dr. McDougall's Digestive Tune-Up*, by John A. McDougall, MD, Healthy Living Publications, 2006.

- *Dr. Neal Barnard's Program for Reversing Diabetes*, by Neal D. Barnard, MD, Rodale, 2007.

- *Everyday Happy Herbivore*, by Lindsay S. Nixon, BenBella Books, 2011.

- *Forks Over Knives—The Cookbook*, by Del Sroufe, The Experiment, 2011.

- *Forks Over Knives: The Plant-Based Way to Health*, by Gene Stone (ed.), The Experiment, 2011.

- *Happy Herbivore Abroad*, by Lindsay S. Nixon, BenBella Books, 2012.

- *Keep It Simple, Keep It Whole*, by Alona Pulde, MD, and Matthew Lederman, MD, Exsalus Health & Wellness Center, 2009.

- *My Beef with Meat*, by Rip Esselstyn, Grand Central Life & Style, 2013.

- *Power Foods for the Brain: An Effective 3-Step Plan to Protect Your Mind and Strengthen Your Memory*, by Neal Barnard, Grand Central Life & Style, 2013.

- *Prevent and Reverse Heart Disease*, by Caldwell B. Esselstyn Jr., MD, Avery Books, 2007.

- *The China Study*, by T. Colin Campbell, PhD, and Thomas M. Campbell II, BenBella Books, 2006.

- *The Engine 2 Diet*, by Rip Esselstyn, Grand Central Books, 2009.

- *The McDougall Program for Maximum Weight Loss*, by John McDougall, MD, Plume, 1995.

- *The McDougall Program: 12 Days to Dynamic Health*, by John A. McDougall, MD, Plume, 1991.

- *The McDougall Quick & Easy Cookbook*, by John A. McDougall, MD, and Mary McDougall, Plume, 1999.

- *The New McDougall Cookbook*, by John McDougall, MD, and Mary McDougall, Plume, 1997.

- *The Pleasure Trap*, by Douglas J. Lisle, PhD, and Alan Goldhamer, DC, Book Publishing Company, 2006.

- *The Starch Solution*, by John A. McDougall, MD, and Mary McDougall, Rodale Books, 2012.

- *Whole, Rethinking the Science of Nutrition*, by T. Colin Campbell, PhD, with Howard Jacobson, PhD, BenBella Books, 2013.

DVDS

- *Forks Over Knives*, Virgil Films and Entertainment, 2011.

- *Forks Over Knives—The Extended Interviews*, Virgil Films and Entertainment, 2013.

- *Losing Weight Without Losing Your Mind*, by Doug Lisle, PhD, John & Mary McDougall Productions, 2007.

- *The Pleasure Trap*, by Doug Lisle, PhD, John & Mary McDougall Productions, 2004.

- *The Willpower Paradox*, by Doug Lisle, PhD, John & Mary McDougall Productions, 2013.

- An assortment of nutrition DVDs available at www.jeffnovick.com

COURSES

- eCornell Certificate in Plant-Based Nutrition: www.nutritionstudies.org

- The Starch Solution Certification Course: www.drmcdougall.com

Notes

1. Alan S. Go, Dariush Mozaffarian, Veronique L. Roger, et al., "Heart Disease and Stroke Statistics—2013 Update: A Report from the American Heart Association," *Circulation* 127 (January 1, 2013): e6–e245; Centers for Disease Control and Prevention, "Heart Disease Facts," 2014, http://www.cdc.gov/heartdisease/facts.htm.

2. American Cancer Society, "Cancer Facts & Figures," 2012, http://www.cancer.org/acs/groups/content/@epidemiologysurveilance/documents/document/acspc-031941.pdf.

3. American Diabetes Association, "Fast Facts: Data & Statistics about Diabetes," 2013, http://professional.diabetes.org/admin/UserFiles/0%20-%20Sean/14_fast_facts_june2014_final3.pdf.

4. Centers for Disease Control and Prevention, "Childhood Obesity Facts," July 2013, http://www.cdc.gov/healthyyouth/obesity/facts.htm.

5. Wenjun Zhong, Hilal Maradit-Kremers, Jennifer L. St. Sauver, et al., "Age and Sex Patterns of Drug Prescribing in a Defined American Population," *Mayo Clinic Proceedings* 88 (July 2013): 687–707.

6. Tina H. T. Chiu, H. Y. Huang, Y. F. Chiu, et al., "Taiwanese Vegetarians and Omnivores: Dietary Composition, Prevalence of Diabetes and IFG," *PLOS One* (February 11, 2014), http://www.plosone.org/article/info%3Adoi%2F10.1371%2F journal.pone.0088547; K. E. Bradbury, F. L. Crowe, P. N. Appleby, J. A. Schmidt, R. C. Travis, and T. J. Key, "Serum Concentrations of Cholesterol, Apolipoprotein A-I and Apolipoprotein B in a Total of 1694 Meat-Eaters, Fish-Eaters, Vegetarians and Vegans," *European Journal of Clinical Nutrition* 68 (February 2014): 178–83; Sylvia H. Ley, Qi Sun, Walter C. Willett et al., "Associations between Red Meat Intake and Biomarkers of Inflammation and Glucose Metabolism in Women," *American Journal of Clinical Nutrition* 99 (February 2014): 352–60; An Pan, Qi Sun, Adam M. Berstein, JoAnn E. Manson, Walter C. Willett, and Frank B. Hu, "Changes in Red Meat Consumption and Subsequent Risk of Type 2 Diabetes Mellitus: Three Cohorts of US Men and Women," *JAMA Internal Medicine* 173 (July 22, 2013): 1328–35; William B. Grant, "A Multicountry Ecological Study of Cancer Incidence Rates in 2008 with Respect to Various Risk-Modifying Factors," *Nutrients* 6 (2014): 163–89; Eunjung Kim, Desire Coelho, and François Blachier, "Review of the Association between Meat Consumption and Risk of Colorectal

Cancer," *Nutrition Research* 33 (December 2013): 983–94; Min-Soo Kim, Seong-Soo Hwang, Eun-Jin Park, and Jin-Woo Bae, "Strict Vegetarian Diet Improves the Risk Factors Associated with Metabolic Diseases by Modulating Gut Microbiota and Reducing Intestinal Inflammation," *Environmental Microbiology Reports* 5 (October 2013): 765–75.

7. Kate Marsh, Carol Zeuschner, and Angela Saunders, "Health Implications of a Vegetarian Diet: A Review," *American Journal of Lifestyle Medicine* 6 (May–June 2012): 250–67.

8. D. Ornish, S. E. Brown, J. H. Billings, et al., "Can Lifestyle Changes Reverse Coronary Heart Disease? The Lifestyle Heart Trial," *Lancet* 336 (July 21, 1990): 129–33.

9. Neal D. Barnard, Joshua Cohen, David J. A. Jenkins, et al., "A Low-Fat Vegan Diet and a Conventional Diabetes Diet in the Treatment of Type 2 Diabetes: A Randomized, Controlled, 74-Week Clinical Trial," *American Journal of Clinical Nutrition* 89 (May 2009): 1588S–96S.

10. Philip J. Tuso, Mohamed H. Ismail, Benjamin P. Ha, and Carole Bartolotto, "Nutritional Update for Physicians: Plant-Based Diets," *The Permanente Journal* 17 (Spring 2013): 61–66.

11. Cheryl L. Rock, Colleen Doyle, Wendy Demark-Wahnefried, et al., "Nutrition and Physical Activity Guidelines for Cancer Survivors," *CA: A Cancer Journal for Clinicians* 62 (July–August, 2012): 243–74.

12. Kate Marsh, Carol Zeuschner, and Angela Saunders, "Health Implications of a Vegetarian Diet: A Review," *American Journal of Lifestyle Medicine* 6 (May–June 2012): 250–67.

13. William B. Grant, "Trends in Diet and Alzheimer's Disease During the Nutrition Transition in Japan and Developing Countries," *Journal of Alzheimer's Disease* 38 (2014): 611–20; M. C. Morris, D. A. Evans, C. C. Tangney, J. L. Bienias, and R. S. Wilson, "Associations of Vegetable and Fruit Consumption with Age-Related Cognitive Change," *Neurology* 67 (October 24, 2006): 1370–76.

14. Lennart Hansson, "Antihypertensive Treatment: Does the J-Curve Exist?" *Cardiovascular Drugs and Therapy* 14 (August 2000): 367–72.

15. Subodh Verma and Marty Strauss, "Angiotensin Receptor Blockers and Myocardial Infarction," *BMJ* 329 (November 25, 2004): 1248–99; Ilke Sipahi, Sara M. Debanne, Douglas Y. Rowland, Daniel I. Simon, and James C. Fang, "Angiotensin-Receptor Blockade and Risk of Cancer: Meta-Analysis of Randomised Controlled Trials," *Lancet Oncology* 11 (July 2010): 627–36; Kenji

Ueshima, Kennichi Fukami, Katsuhiko Hiramori, et al., "Is Angiotensin-Converting Enzyme Inhibitor Useful in a Japanese Population for Secondary Prevention after Acute Myocardial Infarction? A Final Report of the Japanese Acute Myocardial Infarction Prospective (JAMP) Study," *American Heart Journal* 148 (August 2004): 292–99; Colleen J. Maxwell, David B. Hogan, and Erika M. Ebly, "Calcium-Channel Blockers and Cognitive Function in Elderly People: Results from the Canadian Study of Health and Aging," *Canadian Medical Association Journal* 161 (September 7, 1999): 501–6; A. B. Beiderbeck-Noll, M. C. J. M. Sturkenboom, P. D. van der Linden, et al. "Verapamil Is Associated with an Increased Risk of Cancer in the Elderly: The Rotterdam Study," *European Journal of Cancer* 39 (January 2003): 98–105; Marco Pahor, Jack M. Guralnik, Luigi Ferrucci, et al., "Calcium-Channel Blockade and Incidence of Cancer in Aged Populations," *Lancet* 348 (August 1996): 493–97; Annette L. Fitzpatrick, Janet R. Daling, Curt D. Furberg, Richard A. Kronmal, and Joel L. Weissfeld, "Use of Calcium Channel Blockers and Breast Carcinoma Risk in Postmenopausal Women," *Cancer* 80 (October 15, 1997): 1438–47.

16. U.S. Food and Drug Administration, "FDA Expands Advice on Statin Risks," January 31, 2014, http://www.fda.gov/forconsumers/consumerupdates/ucm293330 .htm; Aleesa A. Carter, Tara Gomes, Ximena Camacho, David N. Juurlink, Baiju R. Shah, and Muhammad M. Mamdani, "Risk of Incident Diabetes among Patients Treated with Statins: Population Based Study," *BMJ* 346 (May 23, 2013); Melinda Wenner Moyer, "It's Not Dementia, It's Your Heart Medication: Cholesterol Drugs and Memory," *Scientific American,* September–October 2010; D. Scott, L. Blizzard, J. Fell, and G. Jones, "Statin Therapy, Muscle Function and Falls Risk in Community-Dwelling Older Adults," *Quarterly Journal of Medicine* 102 (2009): 625–33; Paul D. Thompson, Priscilla Clarkson, and Richard H. Karas, "Statin-Associated Myopathy," *Journal of the American Medical Association* 289 (April 2, 2003): 1681–90; Naveed Sattar, David Preiss, Heather M. Murray, et al., "Statins and Risk of Incident Diabetes—A Collaborative Meta-Analysis of Randomised Statin Trials," *Lancet* 375 (February 2010): 735–42.

17. Mark F. Newman, Jerry L. Kirchner, Barbara Phillips-Bute, et al., "Longitudinal Assessment of Neurocognitive Function after Coronary-Artery Bypass Surgery," *New England Journal of Medicine* 344 (February 8, 2001): 395–402.

18. Steven E. Nissen and Kathy Wolski, "Effect of Rosiglitazone on the Risk of Myocardial Infarction and Death from Cardiovascular Causes," *New England Journal of Medicine* 356 (June 14, 2007): 2457–71; Andrea L. C. Schneider, Emma K. Williams, Frederick L. Brancati, Saul Blecker, Josef Coresh, and Elizabeth Selvin,

"Diabetes and Risk of Fracture-Related Hospitalization: The Atherosclerosis Risk in Communities Study," *Diabetes Care* 36 (May 2013): 1153–58; Stephanie Saul, "Heart Attack Risk Seen in Drug for Diabetes," *New York Times,* May 22, 2007, http://www.nytimes.com/2007/05/22/business/22drug.html?pagewanted=all&_r=0; Ioanna Tzoulaki, Mariam Molokhia, Vasa Curcin, et al., "Risk of Cardiovascular Disease and All Cause Mortality among Patients with Type 2 Diabetes Prescribed Oral Antidiabetes Drugs: Retrospective Cohort Study using UK General Practice Research Database," *BMJ* 339 (December 4, 2009): b4731.

19. Edwin Rock and Angela DeMichele, "Nutritional Approaches to Late Toxicities of Adjuvant Chemotherapy in Breast Cancer Survivors," *Journal of Nutrition* 133 (November 2003): 3785S–93S, https://www.bcm.edu/healthcare/care-centers/breast-care-center/patient-information/treatment-medications-side-effects/chemotherapy.

20. Anthony B. Miller, Claus Wall, Cornelia J. Baines, Ping Sun, Teresa To, and Steven A. Narod, "Twenty-five Year Follow-up for Breast Cancer Incidence and Mortality of the Canadian National Breast Screening Study: Randomised Screening Trial," *BMJ* 348 (February 11, 2014): g366; H. Gilbert Welch, "Mammograms Can Help—and Harm," CNN Opinion, November 20, 2013, www.cnn.com/2013/11/20/opinion/welch-mammogram-robach; H. Gilbert Welch and Honor J. Passow, "Quantifying the Benefits and Harms of Screening Mammography," *JAMA Internal Medicine* 174 (March 2014): 448–54; Archie Bleyer and H. Gilbert Welch, "Effect of Three Decades of Screening Mammography on Breast-Cancer Incidence," *New England Journal of Medicine* 367 (November 22, 2012): 1998–2005.

21. "Bone-Density Tests: When You Need Them—and When You Don't," Choosing Wisely, Consumer Reports Health, May 2012, www.choosingwisely.org/doctor-patient-lists/bone-density-tests; Deborah Marshall, Olof Johnell, and Hans Wedel, "Meta-Analysis of How Well Measures of Bone Mineral Density Predict Occurrence of Osteoporotic Fractures," *BMJ* 312 (May 18, 1996): 1254–59; Terence J. Wilkin, "Changing Perceptions in Osteoporosis," *BMJ* 318 (1999): 862–64; Angela Cheung and Allan S. Detsky, "Osteoporosis and Fractures: Missing the Bridge?" *Journal of the American Medical Association* 26 (March 26, 2008): 1468–70; Terence J. Wilkin and Devasenan Devendra, "For and Against: Bone Densitometry Is Not a Good Predictor of Hip Fracture," *BMJ* 323 (October 6, 2001): 795–99; Therapeutics Initiative, "A Systematic Review of the Harms of Biphosphonates," *Therapeutics Letter,* no. 84 (November–December 2011), http://www.ti.ubc.ca/letter84.

22. Fritz H. Schröder, Jonas Hugosson, Monique J. Roobol, et al., "Screening and Prostate-Cancer Mortality in a Randomized European Study," *New England*

Journal of Medicine 360 (March 26, 2009): 1320–28; Gerald L. Andriole, David Crawford, Robert L. Grubb, et al., "Mortality Results from a Randomized Prostate-Cancer Screening Trial," *New England Journal of Medicine* 360 (March 26, 2009): 1310–19; Ruth Etzioni, David F. Penson, Julie M. Legler, et al., "Overdiagnosis Due to Prostate-Specific Antigen Screening: Lessons from U.S. Prostate Cancer Incidence Trends," *Journal of the National Cancer Institute* 94 (July 3, 2002): 981–90; Bret T. Howrey, Yong-Fang Kuo, Yu-Li Lin, and James S. Goodwin, "The Impact of PSA Screening on Prostate Cancer Mortality and Overdiagnosis of Prostate Cancer in the United States," *Journal of Gerontology Series A: Biological Sciences and Medical Sciences* 68 (January 2013): 56–61.

23. Jun-Yao Li, Be-Qi Llu, Uang-Yi Li, Zhi-Jian Chen, Xiu-Di Sun, and Shou-De Rong, "Atlas of Cancer Mortality in the People's Republic of China. An Aid for Cancer Control and Research," *International Journal of Epidemiology* 10 (June 1981): 127–33.

24. Junshi Chen, T. Colin Campbell, Junyao Li, and Richard Peto, eds., *Diet, Life-Style and Mortality in China: A Study of the Characteristics of 65 Chinese Counties* (Oxford: Oxford University Press; Ithaca, NY: Cornell University Press; People's Republic of China: People's Medical Publishing House, 1990); T. Colin Campbell and Thomas M. Campbell II, *The China Study: The Most Comprehensive Study of Nutrition Ever Conducted and the Startling Implications for Diet, Weight Loss, and Long-Term Health* (Dallas, TX: BenBella Books, Inc., 2005), 69–79.

25. Richard Doll and Richard Peto, "The Causes of Cancer: Quantitative Estimates of Avoidable Risks of Cancer in the United States Today," *Journal of the National Cancer Institute* 66 (June 1981): 1192–1308.

26. Data from www.cronometer.com using data compiled from the following databases: Nutrition Coordinating Center Food & Nutrient Database, United States Department of Agriculture National Nutrient Database for Standard Reference, the Canadian Nutrient File, and the Irish Food Composition Database.

27. Jaakko Mursu, Kim Robien, Lisa J. Harnack, Kyong Park, and David R. Jacobs, "Dietary Supplements and Mortality Rate in Older Women. The Iowa Women's Health Study," *Archives of Internal Medicine* 171 (October 10, 2011): 1625–33.

28. Stephen P. Fortmann, Brittany U. Burda, Caitlyn A. Senger, Jennifer S. Lin, and Evelyn P. Whitlock, "Vitamin and Mineral Supplements in the Primary Prevention of Cardiovascular Disease and Cancer: An Updated Systematic Evidence Review for the U.S. Preventive Services Task Force," *Annals of Internal Medicine* 159 (December 17, 2013): 824–34.

29. Goran Bjelakovic, Dimitrinka Nikolova, Lise Lotte Gluud, Rosa G. Simonetti, and Christian Gluud, "Mortality in Randomized Trials of Antioxidant Supplements for Primary and Secondary Prevention: Systematic Review and Meta-Analysis," *Journal of the American Medical Association* 297 (February 28, 2007): 842–57.

30. Marijke van Dusseldorp, Jorn Schneede, Helga Refsum, et al., "Risk of Persistent Cobalamin Deficiency in Adolescents Fed a Macrobiotic Diet in Early Life," *American Journal of Clinical Nutrition* 69 (April 1999): 664–71.

31. Michal L. Melamed, Erin D. Michos, Wendy Post, and Brad Astor, "25-Hydroxyvitamin D Levels and the Risk of Mortality in the General Population," *Archives of Internal Medicine* 168 (August 11–25, 2008): 1629–37; Michael F. Holick, "Vitamin D: Importance in the Prevention of Cancers, Type 1 Diabetes, Heart Disease, and Osteoporosis," *American Journal of Clinical Nutrition* 79, no. 3 (March 2004): 362–71.

32. Shia T. Kent, Leslie A. McClure, William L. Crosson, Donna K. Arnett, Virginia G. Wadley, and Nalini Sathiakumar, "Effect of Sunlight Exposure on Cognitive Function among Depressed and Non-depressed Participants: A REGARDS Cross-sectional Study," *Environmental Health* 8 (July 28, 2009): 34.

33. Patty Nelemans, H. Groenendal L. A. Kiemeney, F. H. Rampen, D. J. Ruiter, and A. L. Verbeek, "Effect of Intermittent Exposure to Sunlight on Melanoma Risk among Indoor Workers and Sun-Sensitive Individuals," *Environmental Health Perspectives* 101 (August 1993): 252–55.

34. Evropi Theodoratou, Ioanna Tzoulaki, Lina Zgaga, and John P. A. Ioannidis, "Vitamin D and Multiple Health Outcomes: Umbrella Review of Systematic Reviews and Meta-Analyses of Observational Studies and Randomised Trials," *BMJ* 348 (April 1, 2014): g2035.

35. Miles D. Witham, "More Evidence Is Needed Before General Supplementation," *BMJ* 336 (June 28, 2008): 1451.

36. Andrew O. Odegaard, Woon-Puay Koh, Kazuko Arakawa, Mimi C. Yu, and Mark A. Pereira, "Soft Drink and Juice Consumption and Risk of Physician-Diagnosed Incident Type 2 Diabetes: The Singapore Chinese Health Study," *American Journal of Epidemiology* 171 (March 15, 2010): 701–8; Shilpa N. Bhupathiraju, An Pan, Vasanti S. Malik, et al., "Caffeinated and Caffeine-Free Beverages and Risk of Type 2 Diabetes," *American Journal of Clinical Nutrition* 97 (January 2013): 155–66; Vasanti S. Malik, Barry M. Popkin, George A. Bray, Jean-Pierre Després, Walter C. Willett, and Frank B. Hu, "Sugar-Sweetened Beverages and Risk of Metabolic Syndrome and Type 2 Diabetes," *Diabetes Care* 33 (November 2010): 2477–83.

37. United States Department of Agriculture, "Tips to Help You Eat Whole Grains," http://www.choosemyplate.gov/food-groups/grains-tips.html.

38. Data from www.cronometer.com using data compiled from the following databases: Nutrition Coordinating Center Food & Nutrient Database, United States Department of Agriculture National Nutrient Database for Standard Reference, The Canadian Nutrient File, and the Irish Food Composition Database.

39. Susan A. New and D. Joe Millward, "Calcium, Protein, and Fruit and Vegetables as Dietary Determinants of Bone Health," *American Journal of Clinical Nutrition* 77 (May 2003): 1340–41; Thomas Remer and Friedrich Manz, "Potential Renal Acid Load of Foods and its Influence on Urine pH," *Journal of the American Dietetic Association* 95 (July 1995): 791–97; Eva Warensjö, Liisa Byberg, Håkan Melhus, et al., "Dietary Calcium Intake and Risk of Fracture and Osteoporosis: Prospective Longitudinal Cohort Study," *BMJ* 342 (May 24, 2011): d1473.

40. Morgan E. Levine, Jorge A. Suarez, Sebastian Brandhorst, et al., "Low Protein Intake Is Associated with a Major Reduction in IGF-1, Cancer, and Overall Mortality in the 65 and Younger but Not Older Population," *Cell Metabolism* 19 (March 4, 2014): 407–17.

41. Patricia C. Gaine, Matthew A. Pikosky, William F. Martin, Douglas R. Bolster, Carl M. Maresh, and Nancy R. Rodriguez, "Level of Dietary Protein Impacts Whole Body Protein Turnover in Trained Males at Rest," *Metabolism Clinical and Experimental* 55 (April 2006): 501–7.

42. D. M. Hegsted, "Calcium and Osteoporosis," *Journal of Nutrition* 116 (July 15, 1986): 2316–19.

43. June M. Chan, Edward Giovannucci, Swen-Olof Andersson, Jonathan Yuen, Hans-Olov Adami, and Alicja Wolk, "Dairy Products, Calcium, Phosphorous, Vitamin D, and Risk of Prostate Cancer (Sweden)," *Cancer Causes & Control* 9 (December 1998): 559–66.

44. Qian Xiao, Rachel A. Murphy, Denise K. Houston, Tamara B. Harris, Wong-Ho Chow, and Yikyung Park, "Dietary and Supplemental Calcium Intake and Cardiovascular Disease Mortality: The National Institutes of Health–AARP Diet and Health Study," *JAMA Internal Medicine* 173 (April 22, 2013): 639–46.

45. Karl Michaëlsson, Håkan Melhus, Eva Warensjö Lemming, Alicja Wolk, and Liisa Byberg, "Long Term Calcium Intake and Rates of All Cause and Cardiovascular Mortality: Community Based Prospective Longitudinal Cohort Study," *BMJ* 346 (February 13, 2013): f228.

46. D. M. Hegsted, "Calcium and Osteoporosis," *Journal of Nutrition* 116 (July 15, 1986): 2316–19.

47. Maren Hegsted, Sally A. Schuette, Michael B. Zemel, and Hellen M. Linkswiler, "Urinary Calcium and Calcium Balance in Young Men as Affected by Level of Protein and Phosphorus Intake," *Journal of Nutrition* 111 (March 1981): 553–62; D. Joe Millward, "The Nutritional Value of Plant-Based Diets in Relation to Human Amino Acid and Protein Requirements," *Proceedings of the Nutritional Society* 58 (May 1999): 249–60; Eric C. Westman, William S. Yancy, Joel S. Edman, Keith F. Tomlin, and Christine E. Perkins, "Effect of 6-Month Adherence to a Very Low Carbohydrate Diet Program," *American Journal of Medicine* 113 (July 2002): 30–36; R. Itoh and Y. Suyama, "Sodium Excretion in Relation to Calcium and Hydroxyproline Excretion in a Healthy Japanese Population," *American Journal of Clinical Nutrition* 63 (May 1996): 735–40.

48. Amy Joy Lanou, "Should Dairy Be Recommended as Part of a Healthy Vegetarian Diet? Counterpoint," *American Journal of Clinical Nutrition* 89 (May 2009): 1638S–42S.

49. Elesa T. Crowley, Lauren T. Williams, Tim K. Roberts, Richard H. Dunstan, and Peter D. Jones, "Does Milk Cause Constipation? A Crossover Diet Trial," *Nutrients* 5, no. 1 (January 22, 2013): 253–66; F. Andiran, S. Dayi, and E. Mete, "Cow's Milk Consumption in Constipation and Anal Fissure in Infants and Young Children," *Journal of Paediatrics and Child Health* 39 (July 2003): 329–31; Johanna T. Dwyer, "Health Aspects of Vegetarian Diets," *American Journal of Clinical Nutrition* 48 (September 1988): 712–38; Giuseppe Iacono, Francesca Cavataio, Giuseppe Montalto, et al., "Intolerance of Cow's Milk and Chronic Constipation in Children," *New England Journal of Medicine* 339 (October 15, 1998): 1100–4; Silvia Daher, Soraia Tahan, Dirceu Solé, et al., "Cow's Milk Protein Intolerance and Chronic Constipation in Children," *Pediatric Allergy and Immunology* 12 (December 2001): 339–42; Warren T. K. Lee, Kin S. Ip, June S. H. Chan, Noel W. M. Lui, and Betty W. Y. Young, "Increased Prevalence of Constipation in Pre-School Children is Attributable to Under-Consumption of Plant Foods: A Community-Based Study," *Journal of Paediatrics and Child Health* 44 (April 2008): 170–75.

50. Li-Qiang Qin, Ka He, and Jia-Ying Xu, "Milk Consumption and Circulating Insulin-like Growth Factor-I Level: A Systematic Literature Review," *International Journal of Food Sciences and Nutrition* 60, no. S7 (January 2009): 330–40.

51. Herbert Yu and Thomas Rohan, "Role of the Insulin-Like Growth Factor Family in Cancer Development and Progression," *Journal of the National Cancer Institute* 92 (September 20, 2000): 1472–89; Bodo C. Melnik and Gerd Schmitz, "Role of Insulin, Insulin-like Growth Factor-1, Hyperglycaemic Food and Milk Consumption

of the Pathogenesis of Acne Vulgaris," *Experimental Dermatology* 10, no. 10 (October 2009): 833–41.

52. Jim Bartley and Susan Read McGlashan, "Does Milk Increase Mucus Production?" *Medical Hypotheses* 74 (April 2010): 732–34; John A. Jenkins, Heimo Breiteneder, and E. N. Clare Mills, "Evolutionary Distance from Human Homologs Reflects Allergenicity of Animal Food Proteins," *Journal of Allergy and Clinical Immunology* 120 (December 2007): 1399–1405; D. C. Heiner, "Respiratory Diseases and Food Allergy," *Annals of Allergy, Asthma & Immunology* 53, no. 6, part 2 (December 1984): 657–64; J. Cant, "Food Allergy in Childhood," *Human Nutrition–Applied Nutrition* 39 (August 1985): 277–93.

53. Suvi M. Vertanen, Esa Läärä, Elina Hyppönen, et al., "Cow's Milk Consumption, HLA-DQB1 Genotype, and Type 1 Diabetes: A Nested Case-Control Study of Siblings of Children with Diabetes," *Diabetes* 49 (June 2000): 912–17; American Academy of Pediatrics Work Group on Cow's Milk Protein and Diabetes Mellitus, "Infant Feeding Practices and Their Possible Relationship to the Etiology of Diabetes Mellitus," *Pediatrics* 94 (November 1, 1994): 752–54; Jukka Karjalainen, Julio M. Martin, Mikael Knip, et al., "A Bovine Albumin Peptide as a Possible Trigger of Insulin-Dependent Diabetes Mellitus," *New England Journal of Medicine* 327 (July 30, 1992): 302–7.

54. Allen S. Levine, Catherine M. Kotz, and Blake A. Gosnell, "Sugars: Hedonic Aspects, Neuroregulation, and Energy Balance," *American Journal of Clinical Nutrition* 78 (October 2003): 834S–42S; Barbara A. Smith, Thomas J. Fillion, and Elliott M. Blass, "Orally Mediated Sources of Calming in 1- to 3-Day-Old Human Infants," *Developmental Psychology* [serial online] 26 (September 1, 1990): 731–37; Elliot M. Blass and Vivian Ciaramitaro, "A New Look at Some Old Mechanisms in Human Newborns: Taste and Tactile Determinants of State, Affect, and Action," *Monographs of the Society of Research in Child Development* 59, no. 1 (1994): i–v, 1–81; Pamela J. Brink, "Addiction to Sugar," *Western Journal of Nursing Research* 15 (June 1993): 280–81.

55. This concept derived from *The Pleasure Trap: Mastering the Hidden Force that Undermines Health & Happiness,* by Douglas J. Lisle and Alan Goldhamer (Summertown, TN: Book Publishing Company, 2006).

56. Philip C. Calder, "N-3 Polyunsaturated Fatty Acids, Inflammation, and Inflammatory Diseases," *American Journal of Clinical Nutrition* 83 (June 2006): 1505S–19S.

57. Jennifer J. Otten, Jennifer Pitzi Hellwig, and Linda D. Meyers, eds., *DRI: Dietary Reference Intakes: The Essential Guide to Nutrient Requirements* (Washington, DC:

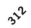

National Academies Press, c. 2006), http://www.nal.usda.gov/fnic/DRI/Essential
_Guide/DRIEssentialGuideNutReq.pdf.

58. B. J. Willcox, D. C. Willcox, H. Todoriki, et al. "Caloric Restriction, the Traditional
Okinawan Diet, and Healthy Aging: The Diet of the World's Longest-Lived People
and Its Potential Impact on Morbidity and Life Span," *Annals of the New York
Academy of Sciences* 1114 (October 2007): 434–55.

59. Antonia Trichopoulou, Tina Costacou, Christina Bamia, and Dimitrios Trichopoulo,
"Adherence to Mediterranean Diet and Survival in a Greek Population," *New
England Journal of Medicine* 348 (June 26, 2003): 2599–608.

60. Ibid.

61. Robert A. Vogel, Mary C. Corretti, and Gary D. Plotnick, "The Postprandial Effect
of Components of the Mediterranean Diet on Endothelial Function," *Journal
of the American College of Cardiology* 36 (November 1, 2000): 1455–60; David H.
Blankenhorn, Ruth L. Johnson, Wendy J. Mack, Hafez A. El Zein, and Laura I. Vailas,
"The Influence of Diet on the Appearance of New Lesions in Human Coronary
Arteries," *Journal of the American Medical Association* 263 (March 23, 1990): 1646–52.

62. D. C. E. Nordström, C. Friman, Y. T. Konttinen, V. E. A. Honkanen, Y. Nasu, and
E. Antila, "Alpha-Linolenic Acid in the Treatment of Rheumatoid Arthritis. A
Double-Blind, Placebo-Controlled and Randomized Study: Flaxseed vs. Safflower
Seed," *Rheumatology International* 14 (1995): 231–34; M. A. Allman, M. M. Pena,
and D. Pang, "Supplementation with Flaxseed Oil Versus Sunflowerseed
Oil in Healthy Young Men Consuming a Low-Fat Diet: Effects on Platelet
Composition and Function," *European Journal of Clinical Nutrition* 49 (March
1995): 169–78; M. R. Namazi, "The Beneficial and Detrimental Effects of Linoleic
Acid on Autoimmune Disorders," *Autoimmunity* 37 (February 2004): 73–75;
P. Purasiri, A. McKechnie, S. D. Heys, and O. Eremin, "Modulation *in Vitro* of
Human Natural Cytotoxicity, Lymphocyte Proliferative Response to Mitogens
and Cytokine Production by Essential Fatty Acids," *Immunology* 92 (October
1997): 166–72; D. Hazlett, "Dietary Fats Appear to Reduce Lung Function,"
Journal of the American Medical Association 223, no. 1 (1973): 15–16; Clifford
W. Welsch, "Relationship Between Dietary Fat and Experimental Mammary
Tumorigenesis: A Review and Critique," *Cancer Research* 52 (April 1992):
2040S–48S; Patrizia Griffini, Olav Fehres, Lars Klieverik, et al., "Dietary Omega-3
Polyunsaturated Fatty Acids Promote Colon Carcinoma Metastasis in Rat Liver,"
Cancer Research 58 (August 1, 1998): 3312–19; Lars Klieverik, Olav Fehres, Patrizia
Griffini, Cornelis J. F. Van Noorden, and Wilma M. Frederiks, "Promotion of

Colon Cancer Metastases in Rat Liver by Fish Oil Diet Is Not Due to Reduced Stroma Formation," *Clinical & Experimental Metastasis* 18 (September 2000): 371–77; Kenneth K. Karroll, "Experimental Evidence of Dietary Factors and Hormone-Dependent Cancers," *Cancer Research* 35 (November 1975): 3374–83; J. H. Weisburger, "Worldwide Prevention of Cancer and Other Chronic Diseases Based on Knowledge of Mechanisms," *Mutation Research* 402 (June 18, 1998): 331–37; Leonard A. Sauer, David E. Blask, and Robert T. Bauchey, "Dietary Factors and Growth and Metabolism in Experimental Tumors," *Journal of Nutritional Biochemistry* 18 (October 2007): 637–49; Clement Ip, "Review of the Effects of Trans Fatty Acids, Oleic Acid, N-3 Polyunsaturated Fatty Acids, and Conjugated Linoleic Acid on Mammary Carcinogenesis in Animals," *American Journal of Clinical Nutrition* 66 (December 1997): 1523S–29S.

63. N. F. Chu, D. Spiegelman, J. Yu, N. Rifai, G. S. Hotamisligil, and E. B. Rimm, "Plasma Leptin Concentrations and Four-Year Weight Gain Among US Men," *International Journal of Obesity and Related Metabolic Disorders* 25 (March 2001): 346–53; N. F. Chu, M. J. Stampfer, D. Spiegelman, N. Rifai, G. S. Hotamisligil, and E. B. Rimm, "Dietary and Lifestyle Factors in Relation to Plasma Leptin Concentrations Among Normal Weight and Overweight Men," *International Journal of Obesity and Related Metabolic Disorders* 25 (January 2001): 106–14; Motonaka Kuroda, Masanori Ohta, Tatsuya Okufuji, et al., "Frequency of Soup Intake and Amount of Dietary Fiber Intake Are Inversely Associated with Plasma Leptin Concentrations in Japanese Adults," *Appetite* 54, no. 3 (June 2010): 538–43.

64. Qi Sun, Donna Spiegelman, Rob M. van Dam, Michelle D. Holmes, Vasanti S. Malik, Walter C. Willett, Frank B. Hu, "White Rice, Brown Rice, and Risk of Type 2 Diabetes in US Men and Women," *Archives of Internal Medicine* 170 (June 14, 2010): 961–69; Guillermo Llanos and Ingrid Libman, "Diabetes in the Americas," *Bulletin of the Pan American Health Organization* 28 (December 1994): 285–301; Teruo Kitagawa Misao Owada, Tatsuhiko Urakami, and Kuniaki Yamauchi, "Increased Incidence of Non-Insulin Dependent Diabetes Mellitus Among Japanese Schoolchildren Correlates with an Increased Intake of Animal Protein and Fat," *Clinical Pediatrics* 37 (February 1998): 111–15; Sok-Ja Janket, JoAnn E. Manson, Howard Sesso, Julie E. Buring, and Simin Liu, "A Prospective Study of Sugar Intake and Risk of Type 2 Diabetes in Women," *Diabetes Care* 26 (April 2003): 1008–15; Lawrence de Koning, Teresa T. Fung, Xiaomei Liao, et al., "Low-Carbohydrate Diet Scores and Risk of Type 2 Diabetes in Men," *American Journal of Clinical Nutrition* 93 (April 2011): 844–50.

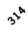

65. Daniel H. Bessesen, "The Role of Carbohydrates in Insulin Resistance," *Journal of Nutrition* 131, no. 10 (October 2001): 2782S–86S; Sok-Ja Janket, JoAnn E. Manson, Howard Sesso, Julie E. Buring, and Simin Liu, "A Prospective Study of Sugar Intake and Risk of Type 2 Diabetes in Women," *Diabetes Care* 26 (April 2003): 1008–15.

66. C. Bolton-Smith and M. Woodward, "Dietary Composition and Fat to Sugar Ratios in Relation to Obesity," *International Journal of Obesity and Related Metabolic Disorders* 18 (December 1994): 820–28; Nicola M. McKeown, Lisa M. Troy, Faul F. Jacques, Udo Hoffmann, Christopher J. O'Donnell and Caroline S. Fox, "Whole- and Refined-Grain Intakes Are Differentially Associated with Abdominal Visceral and Subcutaneous Adiposity in Healthy Adults: The Framingham Heart Study," *American Journal of Clinical Nutrition* 92 (November 2010): 1165–71; Roger L. Hammer, Carol A. Barrier, Elmo S. Roundy, Jeanne M. Bradford, and A. Garth Fisher, "Calorie-Restricted Low-Fat Diet and Exercise in Obese Women," *American Journal of Clinical Nutrition* 49 (January 1989): 77–85; Nick Rose, Kathy Hosig, Brenda Davy, Elena Serrano, and Linda Davis, "Whole-Grain Intake Is Associated with Body Mass Index in College Students," *Journal of Nutrition Education and Behavior* 39 (March–April 2007): 90–94; Kathrine J. Vinknes, Stefan de Vogel, Amany K. Elshorbagy, et al., "Dietary Intake of Protein Is Positively Associated with Percent Body Fat in Middle-Aged and Older Adults," *Journal of Nutrition* 141 (March 2011): 440–46.

67. Roger L. Hammer, Carol A. Barrier, Elmo S. Roundy, Jeanne M. Bradford, and A. Garth Fisher, "Calorie-Restricted Low-Fat Diet and Exercise in Obese Women," *American Journal of Clinical Nutrition* 49 (January 1989): 77–85.

68. George H. Perry, Nathaniel J. Dominy, Katrina G. Claw, et al., "Diet and the Evolution of Human Amylase Gene Copy Number Variation," *Nature Genetics* 39 (October 2007): 1256–60.

69. P. De Feo, C. Di Loreto, P. Lucidi, et al., "Metabolic Response to Exercise," *Journal of Endocrinological Investigation* 26 (September 2003): 851–54; John Temesi, Nathan A. Johnson, Jacqueline Raymond, Catriona A. Burdon, and Helen T. O'Connor, "Carbohydrate Ingestion During Endurance Exercise Improves Performance in Adults," *Journal of Nutrition* 141 (May 2001): 890–97; Patricia C. Gaine, Matthew A. Pikosky, William F. Martin, Douglas R. Bolster, Carl M. Maresh, and Nancy R. Rodriguez, "Level of Dietary Protein Impacts Whole Body Protein Turnover in Trained Males at Rest," *Metabolism Clinical and Experimental* 55 (April 2006): 501–7; American College of Sports Medicine, American Dietetic Association, Dietitians of Canada, "Joint Position Statement: Nutrition and Athletic Performance," *Medicine & Science in Sports & Exercise* 32 (December 2000): 2130–45.

70. Dawn Marks, Allan D. Marks, and Colleen M. Smith, *Basic Medical Biochemistry: A Clinical Approach* (Baltimore, Md: Williams & Wilkins, 1996).

71. Yikyung Park, Amy F. Subar, Albert Hollenbeck, and Arthur Schatzkin, "Dietary Fiber Intake and Mortality in the NIH-AARP Diet and Health Study," *Archives of Internal Medicine* 171 (June 27, 2011): 1061–68; Leah B. Sansbury, Kay Wanke, Paul S. Albert, et al., "The Effect of Strict Adherence to a High-Fiber, High-Fruit and -Vegetable, and Low-Fat Eating Pattern on Adenoma Recurrence," *American Journal of Epidemiology* 170 (September 1, 2009): 576–84; Hope R. Ferdowsian and Neal D. Barnard, "Effects of Plant-Based Diets on Plasma Lipids," *American Journal of Cardiology* 104 (October 1, 2009): 947–56; M. Segasothy and P. A. Phillips, "Vegetarian Diet: Panacea for Modern Lifestyle Diseases?" *QJM* 92 (September 1999): 531–44; John A. Baron, "Dietary Fiber and Colorectal Cancer: An Ongoing Saga," *Journal of the American Medical Association* 294 (December 14, 2005): 2904–6; Voker Mai, Andrew Flood, Ulrike Peters, James V. Lacey, Jr., Catherine Schairer, and Arthur Schatzkin, "Dietary Fibre and Risk of Colorectal Cancer in the Breast Cancer Detection Demonstration Project (BCDDP) Follow-up Cohort," *International Journal of Epidemiology* 32 (April 2003): 234–39; Yikyung Park, David J. Hunter, Donna Spiegelman, et al., "Dietary Fiber Intake and Risk of Colorectal Cancer: A Pooled Analysis of Prospective Cohort Studies," *Journal of the American Medical Association* 294 (December 14, 2005): 2849–57; Tae G. Kiehm, James W. Anderson, and Kyleen Ward, "Beneficial Effects of a High Carbohydrate, High Fiber Diet on Hyperglycemic Diabetic Men," *American Journal of Clinical Nutrition* 29 (August 1976): 895–99; Celia J. Prynne, Aine McCarron. Michael E. J. Wadsworth, and Alison M. Stephen, "Dietary Fibre and Phytate—A Balancing Act: Results from Three Time Points in a British Birth Cohort," *British Journal of Nutrition* 103, no. 2 (January 2010): 274–80; C. J. North, C. S. Venter, and J. C. Jerling, "The Effects of Dietary Fibre on C-Reactive Protein, an Inflammation Marker Predicting Cardiovascular Disease," *European Journal of Clinical Nutrition* 63 (August 2009): 921–33; P. Buil-Cosiales, P. Irimia, E. Ros, et al., "Dietary Fibre Intake Is Inversely Associated with Carotid Intima-Media Thickness: A Cross-Sectional Assessment in the PREDIMED Study," *European Journal of Clinical Nutrition* 63 (October 2009): 1213–19.

72. M. K. Hellerstein, "De Novo Lipogenesis in Humans: Metabolic and Regulatory Aspects," *European Journal of Clinical Nutrition* 53, suppl. 1 (April 1999): 53S–65S; Kevin J. Acheson, Yves Schutz, Thierry Bessard, Krishna Anantharaman, Jean-Pierre Flatt, and Eric Jéquier, "Glycogen Storage Capacity and De Novo Lipogenesis During Massive Carbohydrate Overfeeding in Man," *American Journal*

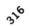

of Clinical Nutrition 48 (August 1988): 240–47; Kaori Minehira, Vincent Bettschart, Hubert Vidal, et al., "Effect of Carbohydrate Overfeeding on Whole Body and Adipose Tissue Metabolism in Humans," *Obesity Research* 11 (September 2003): 1096–1103; Regina M. McDevitt, Sarah J. Bott, Marilyn Harding, W. Andrew Coward, Leslie J. Bluck, and Andrew M. Prentice, "De Novo Lipogenesis During Controlled Overfeeding with Sucrose or Glucose in Lean and Obese Women," *American Journal of Clinical Nutrition* 74 (December 2001): 737–46.

73. Data from www.cronometer.com using data compiled from the following databases: Nutrition Coordinating Center Food & Nutrient Database, United States Department of Agriculture National Nutrient Database for Standard Reference, the Canadian Nutrient File, and the Irish Food Composition Database.

74. A. Britton, M. G. Marmot, and M. Shipley, "Who Benefits Most from the Cardioprotective Properties of Alcohol Consumption—Health Freaks or Couch Potatoes?" *Journal of Epidemiology & Community Health* 62 (October 2008): 905–8.

75. V. Bagnardi, M. Rota, E. Botteri, et al., "Light Alcohol Drinking and Cancer: A Meta-Analysis," *Annals of Oncology* 24 (February 2013): 301–8; Wendy Y. Chen, Bernard Rosner, Susan E. Hankinson, Graham A. Colditz, and Walter C. Willett, "Moderate Alcohol Consumption During Adult Life, Drinking Patterns, and Breast Cancer Risk," *Journal of the American Medical Association* 306 (November 2, 2011): 1884–90.

76. Marilyn L. Kwan, Lawrence H. Kushi, Erin Weltzien, et al., "Alcohol Consumption and Breast Cancer Recurrence and Survival Among Women with Early-Stage Breast Cancer: The Life after Cancer Epidemiology Study," *Journal of Clinical Oncology* 28 (October 10, 2010): 4410–16.

77. S. Goya Wannamethee and A. Gerald Shaper, "Alcohol, Body Weight, and Weight Gain in Middle-aged Men," *American Journal of Clinical Nutrition* 77 (May 2003): 1312–17.

78. S. Bellentani, G. Saccoccio, G. Costa, et al., "Drinking Habits as Cofactors of Risk for Alcohol-Induced Liver Damage," *Gut* 41 (December 1997): 845–50.

79. Markku Kumpari and Pekka Koskinen, "Alcohol, Cardiac Arrhythmias, and Sudden Death," in *Novartis Foundation Symposium 216—Alcohol and Cardiovascular Diseases,* Derek J. Chadwick and Jamie A. Goode, eds. (Chichester, UK: John Wiley, 2007) 68–79; Alvaro Urbano-Márquez and Joaquim Fernández-Solà, "Effects of Alcohol on Skeletal and Cardiac Muscle," *Muscle & Nerve* 30 (December 2004): 689–707.

80. Rohit Loomba, Hwai-I Yang, Jun Su, et al., "Synergism between Obesity and Alcohol in Increasing the Risk of Hepatocellular Carcinoma: A Prospective Cohort Study," *American Journal of Epidemiology* 177 (February 15, 2013): 333–42.

Index

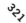

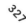

About the Authors

Alona Pulde, MD, is a family practitioner specializing in nutrition and lifestyle medicine in Los Angeles. She received her bachelors of science in biochemistry at UCLA, her masters degree in traditional Oriental medicine from Emperor's College in Southern California, and her doctor of medicine degree from Albany Medical College. Alona developed the lifestyle change program used for patients in the film *Forks Over Knives*, as well as in her clinic, Transition to Health: Medical, Nutrition, and Wellness Center. She is lead author of the book *Keep It Simple, Keep It Whole: Your Guide to Optimum Health*. Alona joined Whole Foods Market in 2010 to serve as a health and wellness medical expert.

Matthew Lederman, MD, is a board-certified internal medicine physician specializing in nutrition and lifestyle medicine. He received his bachelors of science in biology at the University of Michigan, where he graduated with distinction. He received his doctor of medicine degree at Temple University School of Medicine, and completed his residency in internal medicine at the University of Colorado Health Sciences Center. He has participated in projects such as lecturing for the eCornell T. Colin Campbell Certificate Program in Plant-Based Nutrition, as well as appeared in the films *Healing Cancer from Inside Out* and *Forks Over Knives*. Along with Alona, he cofounded Transition to Health: Medical, Nutrition, and Wellness Center and coauthored *Keep It Simple, Keep It Whole*. Matt joined Whole Foods Market in 2010 to help oversee various health and wellness projects.

More from

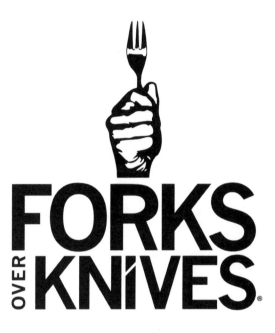

On whole-food, plant-based eating!

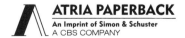

ATRIA PAPERBACK
An Imprint of Simon & Schuster
A CBS COMPANY

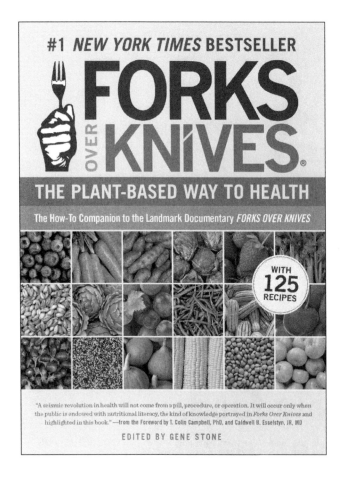

Over 300 recipes for whole-food, plant-based eating all through the year— a *New York Times* bestseller!

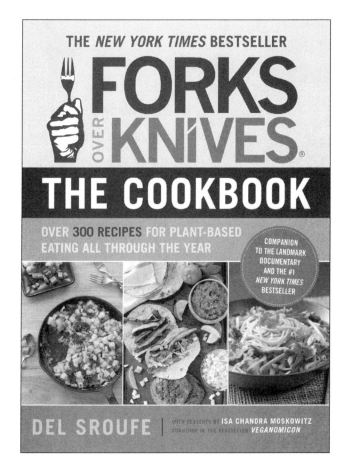

A cookbook with Chef Del Sroufe and his collaborators Julieanna Hever, Judy Micklewright, Isa Chandra Moskowitz, and Darshana Thacker puts the power of real, healthy food in your hands.

• 300 recipes for every meal of the day that transform wholesome fruits, vegetables, grains, and legumes

• Chapters on Breakfasts; Salads, Soups, and Stews; Pasta and Noodles; Stir-fried, Grilled, and Hashed Vegetables; The Amazing Bean; Great Grains; Desserts; and much more

• Cooking the Forks Over Knives way is simple, affordable, and delicious

"*Forks Over Knives* meals are good for the body—and the pocketbook."
—*Indianapolis Star*

Pick up or download your copy today!

Every parent's guide to raising healthy happy kids on a whole-food, plant-based diet.

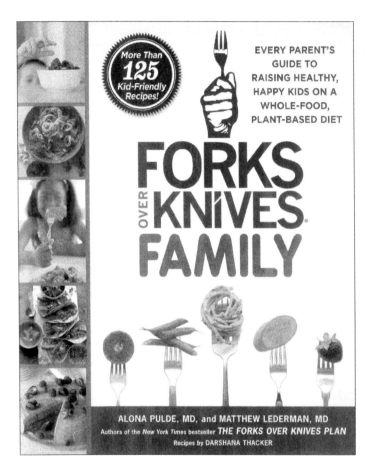
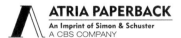

MORE FROM

FORKS OVER KNIVES®

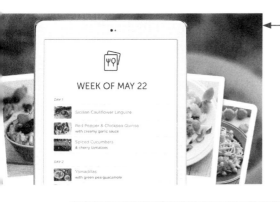

FORKS MEAL
planner

TAKE THE GUESSWORK OUT OF WHAT TO COOK
with our weekly meal plans. Great ideas for easy, healthy,
and low-cost meals.

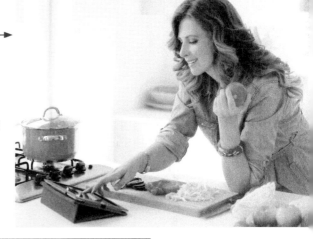

ONLINE COOKING
course

THIS 90-DAY IMMERSIVE ONLINE COOKING COURSE
will teach you all the techniques and styles for how to cook
delicious plant-based meals—all from your own kitchen.

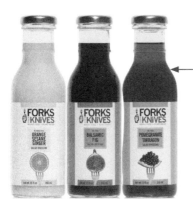

OIL-FREE VEGAN
salad dressings

A PERFECT SALAD is now as easy as a toss and
a pour. These delicious dressings will take your
salads to the next level.

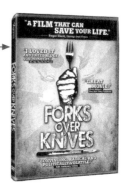

AWARD-WINNING
documentary

THE FILM THAT MADE THE SCIENCE-BACKED case that modern
diseases can be halted or reversed with a whole-food, plant-based diet—
and that helped ignite a food-as-medicine revolution.

forksoverknives.com